SpringerBriefs in Materials

Series Editors

Sujata K. Bhatia, University of Delaware, Newark, USA

Alain Diebold, Schenectady, USA

Juejun Hu, Department of Materials Science and Engineering, Massachusetts Institute of Technology, Cambridge, USA

Kannan M. Krishnan, University of Washington, Seattle, USA

Dario Narducci, Department of Materials Science, University of Milano Bicocca, Milano, Italy

Suprakas Sinha Ray, Centre for Nanostructures Materials, Council for Scientific and Industrial Research, Brummeria, Pretoria, South Africa

Gerhard Wilde, Altenberge, Germany

The SpringerBriefs Series in Materials presents highly relevant, concise monographs on a wide range of topics covering fundamental advances and new applications in the field. Areas of interest include topical information on innovative, structural and functional materials and composites as well as fundamental principles, physical properties, materials theory and design. **Indexed in Scopus (2022).**

SpringerBriefs present succinct summaries of cutting-edge research and practical applications across a wide spectrum of fields. Featuring compact volumes of 50 to 125 pages, the series covers a range of content from professional to academic. Typical topics might include

- A timely report of state-of-the art analytical techniques
- A bridge between new research results, as published in journal articles, and a contextual literature review
- A snapshot of a hot or emerging topic
- An in-depth case study or clinical example
- A presentation of core concepts that students must understand in order to make independent contributions

Briefs are characterized by fast, global electronic dissemination, standard publishing contracts, standardized manuscript preparation and formatting guidelines, and expedited production schedules.

VP Muhammad Rabeeh · T Hanas

Biodegradable Iron Implants: Development, Processing, and Applications

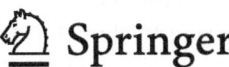 Springer

VP Muhammad Rabeeh
Dr. Moopen's iNEST, Dr. Moopen's
Medical College
Wayanad, Kerala, India

T Hanas
Department of Materials Science
and Engineering
National Institute of Technology Calicut
Kozhikode, Kerala, India

ISSN 2192-1091   ISSN 2192-1105 (electronic)
SpringerBriefs in Materials
ISBN 978-3-031-82098-4   ISBN 978-3-031-82099-1 (eBook)
https://doi.org/10.1007/978-3-031-82099-1

Preface

Recent advancements in biomaterials have led to the emergence of biodegradable metals as a novel alternative for temporary implant applications. Iron-based materials have attracted considerable interest due to their superior mechanical characteristics, biocompatibility, and degradability, making them viable choices for orthopedic, cardiovascular, and other biomedical applications.

This book is dedicated to providing an in-depth investigation of biodegradable iron implant development. It encompasses a broad spectrum of subjects, including the essential characteristics of iron-based degradable materials, their manufacturing methods, processing methods, and surface modification techniques. Readers will find detailed discussions on alloying, surface coatings, and hybrid material systems aimed at enhancing both the bioactivity and mechanical integrity of these implants.

A primary issue in the development of biodegradable iron implants is tailoring the degradation rate to provide safe, predictable degradation within the body, while avoiding the production of detrimental byproducts. Moreover, the mechanical performance of the implant must be adequate throughout the healing period. This book elucidates the essential scientific principles while showcasing the most recent technology advancements propelling progress in this domain, transitioning from laboratory research to clinical applications.

As a researcher engaged in this dynamic and evolving area, I have had the privilege of observing the interdisciplinary collaboration of scientists, engineers, and clinicians who are working tirelessly to bridge the gap between scientific discovery and practical healthcare solutions. I hope that this book will serve as a valuable resource for both early-career researchers and experienced professionals, providing key insights and fostering future innovations in biodegradable iron implants.

I would like to express my deep gratitude to my Ph.D. supervisor, Dr. T. Hanas, from the National Institute of Technology Calicut, as well as to my colleagues and mentors at Dr. Moopen's Medical College, Wayanad, and the National Institute of Technology Calicut, who have supported and guided me throughout this journey. Their invaluable assistance and unwavering commitment have been instrumental in advancing my research endeavors on iron-based biomaterials. I dedicate this book to them with profound respect and appreciation.

Wayanad, India   VP Muhammad Rabeeh
2024

Acknowledgments

Writing this book has been a journey filled with invaluable support, guidance, and inspiration from many people. I am immensely grateful to everyone who has contributed in one way or another to the realization of this work.

First and foremost, I would like to thank my mentors and colleagues, whose wisdom, encouragement, and insights have been pivotal to my professional and personal growth. Dr. Hanas T., my Ph.D. supervisor, has been a constant source of support and inspiration throughout my academic and research career. I am deeply indebted to him for his guidance, which laid the foundation for my research journey and inspired much of the content in this book.

I am also grateful to my colleagues and collaborators at Dr. Moopen's Medical College, whose support has greatly enriched this work. Special thanks to the team at the National Institute of Technology Calicut, who offered guidance and resources that were instrumental during the manuscript preparation.

I would like to acknowledge the AI tools such as ChatGPT, Grammarly, and QuillBot, which significantly contributed to refining the grammar and language during the preparation of this book. This help has been instrumental in ensuring clarity and readability.

Finally, to the readers and the wider scientific community—your dedication to knowledge and innovation drives my passion for research and writing. I hope this book serves as a meaningful contribution to our collective endeavor to understand and advance the field of biomaterials for a better future.

Thank you all for being part of this journey.

VP Muhammad Rabeeh

Contents

Acronyms/Abbreviations

AM	Additive manufacturing
ASTM	American Society for Testing and Materials
BM	Biodegradable metals
CaP	Calcium phosphate
CNT	Carbon nanotubes
Co-Cr	Cobalt-Chromium
CS	Calcium Silicate
DMP	Direct Metal Printing
EDS	Energy dispersive X-ray analysis
E-Fe	Electroformed Fe
EIS	Electrochemical Impedance Spectroscopy
FDA	Food and Drug Administration
$Fe(OH)_2$	Ferrous hydroxide
$Fe(OH)_3$	Ferric hydroxide
H_2	Hydrogen
HA	Hydroxyapatite
HBSS	Hank's balanced salt solution
HV	Vickers hardness
IDP	Insoluble degradation products
ISO	International Organization for Standardization
LPBF	Laser powder bed fusion
MTT	(3-(4,5-dimethylthiazolyl-2)-2, 5-diphenyltetrazolium bromide)
nHA	Nano hydroxyapatite
OCP	Open circuit potential
PBS	Phosphate-buffered saline
PDP	Potentiodynamic polarization
PGA	Polyglycolic acid
PLA	Polylactic acid
PLGA	Poly-lactic-co-glycolic acid
PLLA	Poly-L-lactic acid
PM	Powder metallurgy

PVA	Polyvinyl alcohol
QALY	Quality-adjusted life-year
SBF	Simulated body fluid
SEM	Scanning electron microscope
SLM	Selective Laser Melting
SS	Stainless steel
TCP	Tri-Calcium phosphate
XPS	X-ray photoelectron spectroscopy
XRD	X-ray diffraction

Chapter 1
Introduction to Biodegradable Metals

1.1 Brief Overview

Implants are specifically engineered to provide support or serve as a substitute for tissue that has been injured or impaired. Permanent implants are designed to remain in the body indefinitely and perform their intended duties, while temporary implants are meant to stay inside the body for a specific period of time. After the tissue is healed or the organ regain its normal function, it is necessary to remove the temporary implant from the site. The removal might be accomplished either by surgical procedures or through the natural deterioration or resorption of the implant within the body's physiological environment. During the healing process, it is anticipated that the implant will degrade or get resorbed at a rate compatible with the tissue growth. There are numerous polymeric and ceramic implants that are capable of undergoing degradation within the human body at desired rates. However, polymers and ceramics find limited use in load-bearing temporary implant applications. Currently, such cases use metallic implants made of materials such as stainless steel, cobalt chromium and titanium alloys. These materials are non-degradable, and when employed for temporary implant applications, they necessitate a second surgical procedure for removal from the site. Such surgeries not only increase the cost of healthcare but also increases the risk of hospital-acquired infections and affects patient's overall health. This prompted the researchers to consider a feasible substitute from the metallic category that can undergo tailored degradation in the physiological environment. The degradation rate must align with the rate of tissue growth, and no detrimental by-products should be generated throughout the degradation process. As a result, based on the studies Magnesium (Mg), Iron (Fe), and Zinc (Zn) based alloys are now considered as candidates for biodegradable metallic implants. Although each of these metals has advantages and disadvantages, none of them have been introduced in the worldwide market thus far. As a result, the physicians are compelled to use traditional permanent metallic elements for load-bearing purposes, which inevitably required subsequent surgical procedures once their intended purpose was fulfilled. It is anticipated that

VP. Md. Rabeeh and T. Hanas, *Biodegradable Iron Implants: Development, Processing, and Applications*, SpringerBriefs in Materials, https://doi.org/10.1007/978-3-031-82099-1_1

by adjusting the rate at which the biocompatible metals degrade, mechanical properties and their interaction with human body can help in overcoming this barrier. This introductory chapter provides a brief overview of the need for biodegradable metals, their essential characteristics, and the various types of biodegradable metals.

1.2   Why Biodegradable Metals?

The invention of 18–8 stainless steel in the late 1920s marked a pivotal breakthrough in addressing corrosion issues in the development and clinical use of implant materials (Hermawan 2012). In the 1930s, bio-inert stainless steels (SS) and cobaltchromium (Co–Cr) alloys were considered for temporary and permanent bone fixation devices as well as joint replacements (Wong and Bronzino 2007; Ansari 2029). By the early 1950s, these biomaterials had clinical acceptance and by in 1980s, the first successful cardiovascular stent made from SS was implanted (Shen et al. 2022).

The present demand for orthopaedic and cardiovascular implants has witnessed a surge owing to a rise in the elderly population, the prevalence of bone and cardiovascular diseases, and an increase in the number of accidents. As per the studies reported by Allied Analytics LLP, it is projected that implants will emerge as the most enticing segment within the medical implants industry in terms of generating income. In accordance with the data, the market value of orthopaedic implants was recorded at 49.4 billion US dollars in the year 2023, and it is projected to witness a substantial increase to 76.4 billion US dollars by the year 2033. (Allied Market Research 2024).

In general, the materials used for implants can be classified as metallic, ceramics and polymers. Different classes of materials possess unique advantages and limitations, and the selection of a specific material for a given application is contingent upon its inherent properties. Table 1.1 summarizes the advantages and disadvantages of different class of materials used for implant applications.

Metallic materials are frequently employed for cardiovascular stents and load-bearing prostheses and devices utilized in the repair of bone fractures, owing to their exceptional mechanical properties (Chen and Thouas 2015; Eliaz 2019). Based on the nature of the implant one can classify the implants as permanent or temporary implants. Permanent implants are meant to stay in the body and continue to perform the intended functions. The primary purpose of these interventions is to reinstate the structural integrity and operational capabilities of compromised bones or joints. Therefore, it is imperative that the permanent implant material exhibits biocompatibility and be inert, while demonstrating favourable mechanical properties, wear resistance, and corrosion resistance. The use of metallic materials, including stainless steel, cobalt-chromium and titanium-based alloys, has been approved by the Food and Drug Administration (FDA) for the purpose of serving as enduring orthopaedic implants. This approval is attributed to the exceptional mechanical characteristics and satisfactory biocompatibility exhibited by these materials. Figure 1.1 illustrates the predominant uses of permanent implant for orthopaedic applications.

Table 1.1 Different classes of materials for Implant applications (Wong et al. 2012)

Material	Advantages	Disadvantages	Examples
Ceramics	Biocompatible Inert Strong in compression	Brittle	Dental implants Orthopaedic implants (some)
Polymers	Resilient Easy to fabricate	Poor mechanical properties Time-dependent deformation (creep: stress relaxation) Degradation	Dental implant Vascular grafts Joint socket (knee, shoulder) Ear, nose Soft tissues in general
Metals	Strong Tough Ductile	Corrosion Density	Joint replacement Dental roots Orthopaedic fixation Stents

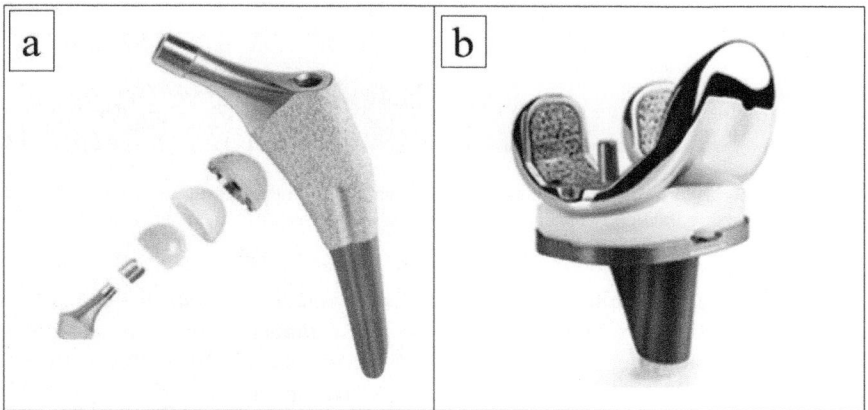

Fig. 1.1 Permanent orthopaedic implants **a** hip joint and **b** knee implant (Adapted with permission of Elsevier from Friis et al. (2017)

A temporary implant or fixation device is designed to be retained within the body for a specific period of time. Once the tissue is healed and is restored, it becomes necessary to remove the temporary implant from the site. Figure 1.2 illustrates various temporary implants use for orthopaedic applications. Currently, most implants used for this function are made of conventional metallic implant materials such as stainless steel (SS), cobalt-chromium (Co–Cr) alloys, and titanium (Ti) alloys (Chen and Thouas 2015).The use of these metallic materials make the implants non degradable and are to be removed by a surgery after the damaged tissue is healed. This second surgery results in additional costs and increased discomfort for the patient, as it involves further medical procedures and recovery time. Moreover, the elastic moduli of bone tissue are far less than those of these conventional implant materials, which leads to stress shielding and, subsequently, decreases stimulus for new bone tissue

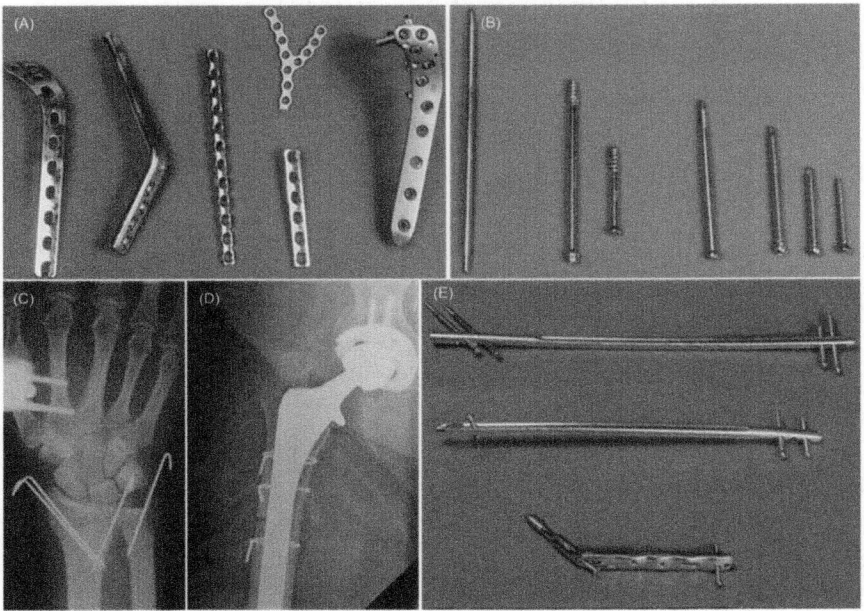

Fig. 1.2 Temporary orthopedic implants **a** Plates, **b** screws, **c** pins, **d** wires, and **e** intramedullary nails used in fracture fixation (Reprinted with permission of Elsevier from Jin and Chu 2019)

growth and bone remodelling resulting in loss of bone density (Nagels et al. 2003; Niinomi et al. 2012). In the case of cardiovascular implants the removal is almost impossible. Thus it is important to have biodegradable metals (BMs) for developing load bearing metallic implants that can degrade and disappear from the implanted site once the desired function is accomplished. These materials are expected to facilitate and support tissue healing before degrading completely at a desired rate. One needs to properly tune the degradation rate of such implants so that the implant removal is compatible with tissue growth. Thus with BMs one will be able to shift approach from "fix—heal—remove" strategy to "fix—heal—disappear" route for temporary implant applications.

1.3 General Requirements of BMs

As mentioned in the previous section the concept of biodegradable metals (BMs) is seen as one of the promising alternatives to avoid removal surgery and stress shielding. BMs are expected to degrade at a predetermined rate in the physiological environment without any harmful effect on tissue, and thereby helps to avoid the second surgery. The implants made of BMs are expected to degrade and disappear

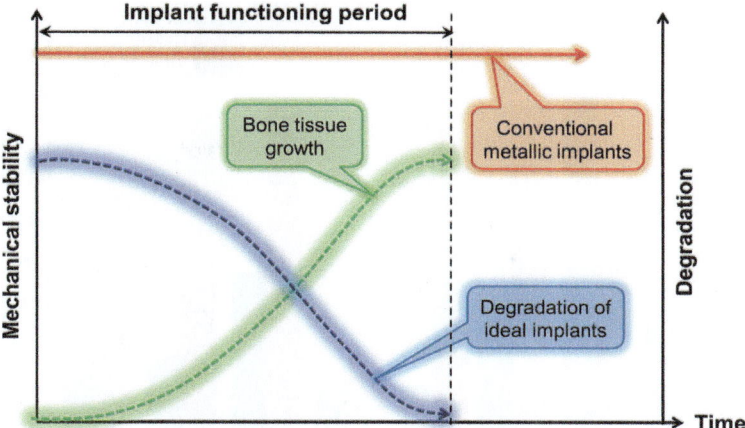

Fig. 1.3 Schematic diagram of degradation behaviour and changes in the mechanical integrity of biodegradable metal implants

from the disease site with little residue (Wong et al. 2012; Li et al. 2014, 2019a; Hermawan 2018). The ideal biodegradable material shall have a desirable degradation rate compatible with the regeneration rate of the tissues. Shuai et al. (2019) reported that the degradation rate of BMs used in bone repair needs to be between 0.2 and 0.5 mmpy depending upon the cases. Nevertheless, the degradation rate will have to conform with the new bone growth rate to ensure the progressive transfer of load to the healing bone and minimise the disadvantages of stress shielding. When the implant degrades, its strength decreases, and the load is progressively transferred to the recovering bone tissue, as shown in Fig. 1.3 (Waizy et al. 2013). The biodegradation of metals inside the body depends primarily on interaction with the physiological environment. Such interaction of some metals can also bring benefits for biomedical applications as reported by Zheng et al. 2014. The BMs can contain vital metallic elements that the human body tissues could gradually absorb and also help in achieving the desired level of degradation (Seal et al. 2009; Zheng et al. 2014). Thus, one can see that the concept of biodegradable metallic implants challenges the conventional paradigm that metallic biomaterials should be resistant to degradation (Bauer et al. 2013) but are required to degrade at the desired rate.

1.4 Types of BMs Materials

Current proposals for degradable metallic biomaterials primarily encompass systems based on magnesium (Mg), zinc (Zn), and iron (Fe). Each of these materials has own advantages and disadvantages. However, no products are successfully launched in the global market so far. Consequently, clinicians are required to rely on traditional,

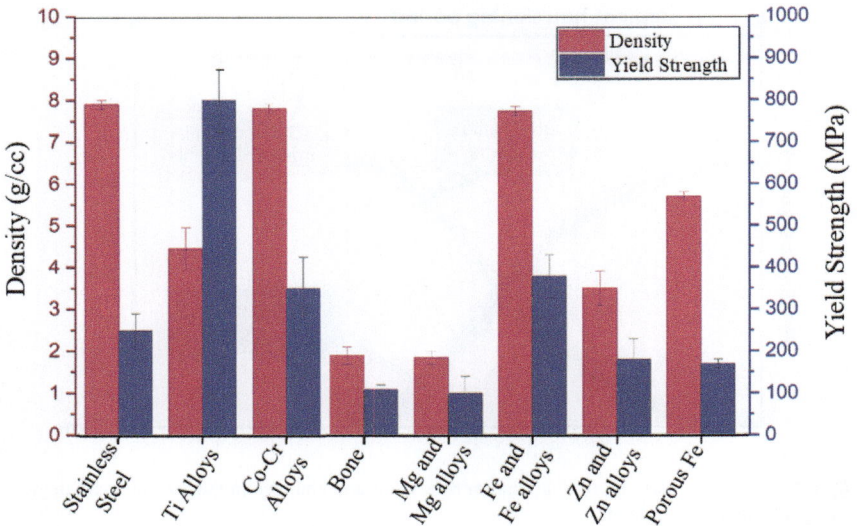

Fig. 1.4 Comparison of mechanical properties of various orthopaedic implant materials

permanent metallic materials for load-bearing applications. Modifying parameters such as the degradation rate, mechanical properties, and the interaction between the implant and surrounding tissue is anticipated to address this issue effectively. Figure 1.4 compares the mechanical properties of various implant metallic materials utilized for orthopedic applications.

1.4.1 Magnesium and Magnesium Alloys

Mg-based alloys have garnered most researched promising biomaterials for degradable implant applications, particularly in the field of orthopedics. Unlike traditional permanent implants composed of materials such as stainless steel or titanium, Mg-based alloys can degrade within the human body, potentially eliminating the need for surgical removal after tissue is healed. One of the key advantages of Mg alloys lies in their mechanical properties, particularly their Young's modulus, which closely aligns with that of human cortical bone. This compatibility makes Mg alloys ideal candidates for load-bearing applications in bone repair and regeneration. Moreover, their biodegradability allows them to be replaced by natural bone over time, a highly desirable characteristic in orthopedic implants. The medical application of Mg was first documented in 1878 when Mg wires were utilized as blood vessel ligatures (Witte (2010)). Since then, various Mg-based devices, such as plates, screws, and connectors, have been explored for use in orthopedic and vascular surgeries. Early applications of Mg-based alloys encountered significant challenges, primarily due to their rapid degradation and variable biocompatibility. Although Mg promotes osteogenesis, its high corrosion rate in physiological environments (ranging from 0.8 to 2.7 mmpy) often resulted in premature implant failure, accompanied by the formation of hydrogen gas pockets and localized tissue irritation (Waizy et al. 2013). Despite these limitations, ongoing research has focused on refining and optimizing Mg alloys to improve their performance in biomedical applications.

Mg-based alloys offer several key advantages, making them attractive candidates for biomedical use. Among these is their excellent biocompatibility, which surpasses that of many synthetic polymers and ceramics. As Mg alloys degrade, they release non-toxic by-products, including Mg ions, which are safely absorbed by the body. These Mg ions have been shown to promote osteogenesis by stimulating bone formation processes, thereby enhancing the osteopromotive properties of Mg alloys (Duan et al. 2020). Additionally, the mechanical properties of Mg alloys closely match those of human bone, reducing the risk of stress shielding—a phenomenon where stronger, non-degradable materials like titanium share almost the full load, leading to the weakening of surrounding bone. Moreover, controlled degradation of Mg alloys can release small quantities of hydrogen gas, which has been found to possess antioxidant properties that reduce post-surgical inflammation (Wang et al 2024).

Despite their advantages, Mg-based alloys face several critical challenges that have hindered their widespread clinical use. The most significant drawback is their rapid degradation in physiological environments, often occurring before the surrounding tissue has fully healed. This premature loss of mechanical integrity can lead to implant failure, compromising the healing process. Additionally, the rapid corrosion of Mg alloys can accumulate and form H_2 gas pockets beneath the skin or in tissue, potentially leading to discomfort or infection. Furthermore, the rapid degradation of Mg alloys limits their application in scenarios that require long-term mechanical stability, such as certain orthopedic or cardiovascular implants.

In response to these challenges, recent research has focused on developing methods to slow the degradation rate of Mg-based alloys through alloying and surface treatments. Alloying Mg with elements such as zinc (Zn), calcium (Ca), and rare earth elements has been shown to enhance corrosion resistance while maintaining biocompatibility and mechanical properties. Additionally, surface treatments such as chemical coatings (e.g., hydroxyapatite, titanium dioxide) and mechanical techniques (e.g., laser shock peening) have been employed to further improve corrosion resistance and mechanical strength. These advancements aim to achieve a balance between the degradation rate of Mg alloys and the tissue healing process, providing sufficient mechanical support during the critical period of healing while minimizing complications associated with rapid corrosion (Istrate et al. 2022).

Mg-based alloys hold significant potential for future medical applications beyond orthopedics, including cardiovascular stents, where biodegradable materials are highly desirable. The development of coatings that enable controlled degradation opens new possibilities for Mg-based implants in areas requiring precise mechanical support over limited time frames. Additionally, research into the anti-inflammatory and anti-cancer properties of Mg further broadens the therapeutic potential of these materials. Although challenges remain, continued advancements in alloy composition, surface treatments, and corrosion control are likely to solidify Mg-based alloys as a viable alternative for a wide range of degradable implant applications in the near future.

1.4.2 Zn and Zn-Based Alloys

Zn-based alloys are emerging as a candidate materials due to their suitability for biodegradable medical implant applications. They exhibit a controlled degradation rate without releasing hydrogen gas, a common issue associated with Mg-based biodegradable metals, making them particularly attractive for use in biomedical environments where excessive gas release lead to complications (Emily Walker 2015; Kabir et al. 2021). Although studies focused on biodegradable metals based on Zn-alloys are relatively new, the potential of Zn was identified long before based on its essential role in various biological processes (Li et al. 2019a). Zinc is a vital element in the body that is critical for numerous enzymatic activities and immune functions. Early studies on Zn alloys for biomedical applications highlighted their moderate degradation rate (typically between 0.1 and 0.3 mm per year), which aligns well with the desired timeframe for tissue healing (Wang et al. 2023). Despite their promising attributes, Zn-based alloys face significant challenges that limit their broader application in medical implants. A major disadvantage is their comparatively poor mechanical strength compared to traditional metals and even magnesium-based alloys. This limitation has restricted their potential use to non-load-bearing applications, such as vascular stents, where requirements on mechanical performance are less stringent (Bryzgalov et al 2024; Istrate et al. 2022). The poor mechanical properties arise from issues such as creep deformation, low-temperature recrystallization, and age hardening, all of which can affect their performance during both storage and clinical use. Furthermore, Zn alloys typically exhibit lower fatigue strength, meaning they cannot withstand the cyclic loading profiles involved in applications like bone fixation. These shortcomings necessitate further research to enhance the strength and stability of Zn-based alloys while retaining their favourable degradation characteristics.

Recent research has focused on alloying Zn with other elements such as magnesium (Mg) and calcium (Ca) to enhance strength and tailor degradation rate in physiological environment. Studies have shown that small additions of alloying elements can improve the mechanical behavior of Zn alloys without compromising their biocompatibility or degradation rate. Additionally, surface modifications such as coating with biocompatible polymers or ceramics are also attempted to further fine-tune the degradation behaviour and preserving mechanical properties (Bryzgalov et al. 2024; Kabir et al. 2021). As research in this area progresses, Zn-based alloys are poised to become a more viable option for a broader range of medical applications, particularly as vascular stents, staples and non-load-bearing orthopedic devices where moderate mechanical strength is sufficient and controlled biodegradability is essential.

1.4.3 Fe and Fe-Based Alloys

Since the early 2000s, Fe-based alloys have been explored as potential biodegradable implant materials. Their exceptional mechanical properties, including high tensile strength and rigidity, make them well-suited for load-bearing applications like orthopedic and cardiovascular devices. The gradual degradation of Fe alloys allows them to maintain structural integrity over an extended period, providing essential mechanical support while tissue regeneration occurs. Early studies demonstrated that Fe alloys exhibit excellent mechanical properties; however, their slow degradation rate in physiological environments posed a challenge. Unlike Mg and Zn-based alloys, which degrade relatively quick in physiological environment, Fe-based systems degrade at rates much slower than the desired for many implant applications. This has led to efforts to accelerate the degradation process while maintaining the inherent mechanical strength of the material. Despite these challenges, Fe alloys continue to be explored for applications where prolonged mechanical stability is critical, such as vascular stents and bone fixation devices (Rabeeh and Hanas 2022; Gorejová et al. 2019; Scarcello and Lison 2020).

One of the primary advantages of Fe-based alloys is their exceptional mechanical strength, which surpasses that of both magnesium and zinc-based biodegradable metals. This makes them particularly suitable for applications requiring long-term load-bearing capacity. Additionally, Fe does not produce hydrogen gas during degradation, a significant advantage over Mg alloys, which can lead to complications due to gas pocket formation (He et al. 2016). However, the slow degradation rate of Fe alloys is a major limitation, as it can lead to prolonged presence in the body beyond the intended support period, potentially causing inflammation or interference with natural tissue regeneration. Furthermore, the high stiffness of Fe alloys can lead to stress shielding, where the implant bears too much load, potentially weakening the bone over time (Ridzwan et al. 2007; He et al. 2016). Also the magnetic nature of the ferroalloy can influence imaging of the implant and diagnosis in patients. To overcome these issues, researchers are investigating various methods to accelerate the corrosion of Fe-based alloys. This includes alloying with elements like manganese (Mn) and palladium (Pd) etc. or applying surface treatments to enhance biodegradation (Heiden et al. 2015, 2016, 2017; Hermawan et al. 2008; Rabeeh and Hanas 2022). These strategies aim to tailor the degradation rate to better match the tissue healing process, making Fe alloys more suitable for a broader range of medical applications. Despite current challenges, Fe-based alloys hold significant potential for use in long-term medical implants, particularly where high mechanical strength is essential and slower degradation is not a drawback.

1.4.4 Comparative Analysis of Mg, Zn, and Fe-Based Biodegradable Metals for Implant Applications

While each material possesses distinct advantages and limitations, a comparative analysis is essential to identify future directions for development. Figure 1.5 depict the degradation of BMs and variations in mechanical integrity during the tissue healing process Mg-based materials, for instance, exhibit a rapid degradation rate in physiological environments, ranging from 0.8 to 2.7 mmpy, while Fe-based systems degrade much more slowly, with rates below 0.2 mmpy (Hermawan et al. 2010; Sing et al. 2015). In contrast, Zn-based biomaterials offer an intermediate degradation rate between 0.1 and 0.3 mmpy, without the release of hydrogen gas, aligning more closely with the desired degradation rates for biodegradable metals (Kabir et al. 2021). However, the mechanical properties of Zn are often low (Table 1.2) for critical medical applications such as stents and orthopedic implants (Vojtěch et al. 2011). Furthermore, Zn and its alloys are prone to issues such as poor fatigue strength, low-temperature recrystallization, creep, and increased susceptibility to natural aging, which can adversely affect the performance of implants during storage and use (Li et al. 2019b).

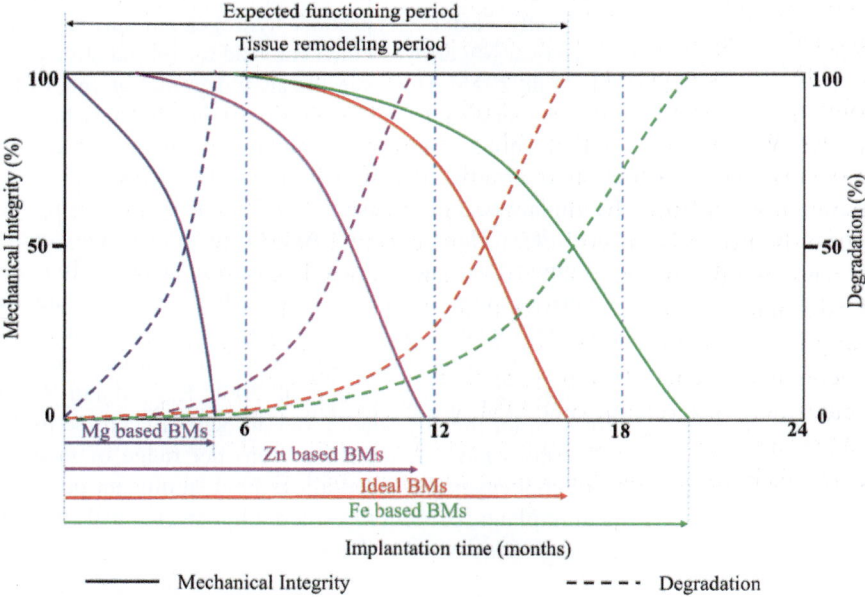

Fig. 1.5 The schematic representation of degradation of BMs and variations in mechanical integrity during the tissue healing process (Reprinted with permission of Springer Nature from Rabeeh and Hanas 2022)

Table 1.2 The mechanical properties of biodegradable metals. (Reprinted from MDPI (CC BY 4.0) (Gąsior et al. 2021)

Material	Yield Strength (MPa)	Young's Modulus (GPa)	Tensile Strength (MPa)	Shear Modulus (GPa)	Elastic Modulus (GPa)	Hardness (HV)
Mg	51	44–45.5	175–235	16–18	44–48	38
Zn	285–325	90–110	90–200	35–45	14–32	42
Fe	108–122	204–212	230–345	78–84	195–235	157

Fe-based systems possess the necessary mechanical properties, good formability, and acceptable biocompatibility for use in medical implants. However, their degradation rate is often too slow, falling below clinical requirements, which can lead to challenges similar to those encountered with conventional, non-biodegradable implant materials. Table 1.3 provides a summary of the key advantages and disadvantages of Mg, Zn, and Fe-based biodegradable metals, highlighting the need for further refinement to optimize their performance in biomedical applications.

Table 1.3 Major advantages and disadvantages of Mg, Zn and Fe-based biodegradable metals. (Reprinted with permission of Springer Nature from Rabeeh and Hanas 2022)

Biodegradable Metal	Advantages	Disadvantages
Mg-based BMs	• Biodegradable • Biocompatible • Can be tuned to promote biomineralisation and osseointegration • Density and elastic modulus close to that of human bone and thereby reduce the chances of stress-shielding • MRI compatible • An essential element for the human body	• Extremely high degradation rate • H_2 gas evolution during degradation • Local rise of pH near the implant site • Poor mechanical strength for load-bearing application • Premature loss of mechanical integrity
Zn-based BMs	• Biodegradable • Acceptable biocompatibility • Good processability • No H_2 gas evolution during degradation • Non-toxic degradation products	• Poor mechanical strength • Proneness to creep • Age hardening
Fe-Based BMs	• Biodegradable • High tensile strength and formability • Acceptable biocompatibility • MRI compatible (in austenitic phase), • No H_2 gas evolution during degradation	• Very low degradation rate • High elastic modulus leads to stress shielding • Non-MRI compatible (in Ferritic phase)

It is critical to consider both the degradation properties and the mechanical characteristics of the implant material. When biodegradable metal is employed in clinical applications, its exceptional strength distinguishes it from other biodegradable polymers, making it an ideal material for load-bearing applications. Iron and its alloys exhibit a combination of strength and ductility with a high elastic module, particularly when compared to magnesium and zinc. Due to the inherent advantages of Fe as a classic engineering material, such as good mechanical characteristics, superior machinability and low cost, they have the potential to be a primary source of biodegradable metallic materials. This book explores metallurgical and surface modifications of Fe-based systems to tailor their biodegradation and bioactivity in physiological environments. It covers the development of biodegradable iron, various manufacturing routes, and key processing techniques, while also examining its potential applications in medical implants.

References

Allied Market Research (2024) Orthopedic implants market size, share & trends analysis report. Retrieved October 31, 2024, from https://www.alliedmarketresearch.com/orthopedic-implants-market

Ansari M (2019) Bone tissue regeneration: biology, strategies and interface studies. Prog Biomater 8:223–237. https://doi.org/10.1007/S40204-019-00125-Z

Bauer S, Schmuki P, von der Mark K, Park J (2013) Engineering biocompatible implant surfaces: Part I: materials and surfaces. Prog Mater Sci 58:261–326

Bryzgalov V, Kistanov AA, Khafizova E et al (2024) Experimental study of corrosion rate supplied with an ab-initio elucidation of corrosion mechanism of biodegradable implants based on Ag-doped Zn alloys. Appl Surf Sci 652:159300. https://doi.org/10.1016/j.apsusc.2024.159300

Chen Q, Thouas GA (2015) Metallic implant biomaterials. Mater Sci Eng R Rep 87:1–57. https://doi.org/10.1016/j.mser.2014.10.001

Duan H, Cao C, Wang X et al (2020) Magnesium-alloy rods reinforced bioglass bone cement composite scaffolds with cortical bone-matching mechanical properties and excellent osteoconductivity for load-bearing bone in vivo regeneration. Sci Rep 10:1–14. https://doi.org/10.1038/s41598-020-75328-7

Eliaz N (2019) Corrosion of metallic biomaterials: a review. Materials 12:407. https://doi.org/10.3390/ma12030407

Emily Walker MH (2015) Magnesium, Iron and Zinc alloys, the trifecta of bioresorbable orthopaedic and vascular implantation—a review. J Biotechnol Biomater 05:178. https://doi.org/10.4172/2155-952X.1000178

Friis EA, Tsao AK, Topoleski LDT, Jones LC (2017) Introduction to mechanical testing of orthopedic implants. In: Friis E (ed) Mechanical testing of orthopaedic implants. Woodhead Publishing, pp 3–15

Gąsior G, Szczepański J, Radtke A (2021) Biodegradable iron-based materials—what was done and what more can be done? Materials 14:3381. https://doi.org/10.3390/ma14123381

Gorejová R, Haverová L, Oriňaková R et al (2019) Recent advancements in Fe-based biodegradable materials for bone repair. J Mater Sci 54:1913–1947. https://doi.org/10.1007/s10853-018-3011-z

He J, He F, Li D et al (2016) Advances in Fe-based biodegradable metallic materials. RSC Adv, 112819–112838.https://doi.org/10.1039/c6ra20594a

Heiden M, Johnson D, Stanciu L (2016) Surface modifications through dealloying of Fe-Mn and Fe-Mn-Zn alloys developed to create tailorable, nanoporous, bioresorbable surfaces. Acta Mater 103:115–127. https://doi.org/10.1016/j.actamat.2015.10.002

Heiden M, Nauman E, Stanciu L (2017) Bioresorbable Fe–Mn and Fe–Mn–HA materials for orthopedic implantation: enhancing degradation through porosity control. Adv Healthc Mater 6:1700120. https://doi.org/10.1002/ADHM.201700120

Heiden M, Walker E, Nauman E, Stanciu L (2015) Evolution of novel bioresorbable iron-manganese implant surfaces and their degradation behaviors in vitro. J Biomed Mater Res A 103:185–193. https://doi.org/10.1002/jbm.a.35155

Hermawan H (2012) Introduction to metallic biomaterials. In: Biodegradable metals from concept to applications, pp 1–11

Hermawan H (2018) Updates on the research and development of absorbable metals for biomedical applications. Prog Biomater 7:93–110. https://doi.org/10.1007/S40204-018-0091-4

Hermawan H, Alamdari H, Mantovani D, Dubé D (2008) Iron–manganese: new class of metallic degradable biomaterials prepared by powder metallurgy. Powder Metall 51:38–45. https://doi.org/10.1179/174329008X284868

Hermawan H, Dubé D, Mantovani D (2010) Degradable metallic biomaterials for cardiovascular applications. In: Metals for biomedical devices. Elsevier Ltd, pp 379–404

Istrate B, Munteanu C, Antoniac I-V, Lupescu Ş-C (2022) Current research studies of Mg–Ca–Zn biodegradable alloys used as orthopedic implants—review. Crystals 12:1468. https://doi.org/10.3390/cryst12101468

Jin W, Chu PK (2019) Orthopedic implants. In: Narayan R (ed) Encyclopedia of biomedical engineering. Elsevier, pp 425–439. https://doi.org/10.1016/B978-0-12-801238-3.10999-7

Kabir H, Munir K, Wen C, Li Y (2021) Recent research and progress of biodegradable zinc alloys and composites for biomedical applications: Biomechanical and biocorrosion perspectives. Bioact Mater 6:836–879. https://doi.org/10.1016/J.BIOACTMAT.2020.09.013

Li C, Guo C, Fitzpatrick V, et al (2019a) Design of biodegradable, implantable devices towards clinical translation. Nat Rev Mater 5:1 5:61–81. https://doi.org/10.1038/s41578-019-0150-z

Li G, Yang H, Zheng Y et al (2019b) Challenges in the use of zinc and its alloys as biodegradable metals: perspective from biomechanical compatibility. Acta Biomater 97:23–45. https://doi.org/10.1016/J.ACTBIO.2019.07.038

Li H, Zheng Y, Qin L (2014) Progress of biodegradable metals. Progress Nat Sci Mater Int 24:414–422

Nagels J, Stokdijk M, Rozing PM (2003) Stress shielding and bone resorption in shoulder arthroplasty. J Shoulder Elbow Surg 12:35–39. https://doi.org/10.1067/mse.2003.22

Niinomi M, Nakai M, Hieda J (2012) Development of new metallic alloys for biomedical applications. Acta Biomater 8:3888–3903. https://doi.org/10.1016/j.actbio.2012.06.037

Rabeeh VPM, Hanas T (2022) Progress in manufacturing and processing of degradable Fe-based implants: a review. Progress Biomater 11:2 11:163–191. https://doi.org/10.1007/S40204-022-00189-4

Ridzwan MIZ, Shuib S, Hassan AY et al (2007) Problem of stress shielding and improvement to the hip implant designs: a review. J Med Sci 7:460–467. https://doi.org/10.3923/JMS.2007.460.467

Scarcello E, Lison D (2020) Are Fe-based stenting materials biocompatible? A critical review of in vitro and in vivo studies. J Funct Biomater 11:2

Seal CK, Vince K, Hodgson MA (2009) Biodegradable surgical implants based on magnesium alloys—A review of current research. IOP Conf Ser Mater Sci Eng 4:012011. https://doi.org/10.1088/1757-899X/4/1/012011

Shen Y, Yu X, Cui J, Yu F, Liu M, Chen Y, Wu J, Sun B, Mo X (2022) Development of biodegradable polymeric stents for the treatment of cardiovascular diseases. Biomolecules 12:1245. https://doi.org/10.3390/biom12091245

Shuai C, Li S, Peng S et al (2019) Biodegradable metallic bone implants. Mater Chem Front 3:544–562

Sing NB, Mostavan A, Hamzah E et al (2015) Degradation behavior of biodegradable Fe35Mn alloy stents. J Biomed Mater Res B Appl Biomater 103:572–577. https://doi.org/10.1002/JBM. B.33242

Vojtěch D, Kubásek J, Šerák J, Novák P (2011) Mechanical and corrosion properties of newly developed biodegradable Zn-based alloys for bone fixation. Acta Biomater 7:3515–3522. https:// doi.org/10.1016/J.ACTBIO.2011.05.008

Wang H, Yang K, Ma Y, Xu L (2023) Research progress on biodegradable Zn-based alloy materials. Am J Life Sci 11:56–63. https://doi.org/10.11648/j.ajls.20231104.12

Wang B, Pan S, Nie C et al (2024) Magnesium implantation as a continuous hydrogen production generator for the treatment of myocardial infarction in rats. Sci Rep 14:10959. https://doi.org/ 10.1038/s41598-024-60609-2

Waizy H, Seitz JM, Reifenrath J et al (2013) Biodegradable magnesium implants for orthopedic applications. J Mater Sci 48:39–50

Witte F (2010) The history of biodegradable magnesium implants: a review. Acta Biomater 6:1680–1692. https://doi.org/10.1016/j.actbio.2010.02.028

Wong JY, Bronzino JD (2007) Biomaterials. CRC Press, Boca Raton, Fla

Wong JY, Bronzino JD, Peterson DR et al (2012) Biomaterials, 1st edn. CRC Press

Zheng YF, Gu XN, Witte F (2014) Biodegradable metals. Mater Sci Eng R Rep 77:1–34

Chapter 2
Iron as Biodegradable Implant

2.1 Fe: A Brief Overview

Iron is a transition metal with the atomic number 26 and is the fourth most prevalent element in the earth's crust (about 5%), represented by the symbol Fe. It exhibits a range of oxidation states (-2 to $+6$), with $+2$ and $+3$ being the most common. Only meteoroids or environments with low oxygen levels can retain elemental or pure iron in nature, as it reacts with oxygen rapidly and forms an exterior passive film. It has good mechanical properties at room temperature, with an elastic modulus of 200 GPa, and a shear modulus of 78 GPa (John E 2011). A major fraction of world's metal alloy manufacturing is based on iron-based systems (Emsley 2011). This high production and use are due to the abundant supply of iron ores, ease of use, comparatively low processing costs, and the vast range of properties available from these alloys.

2.2 History of Fe as an Implant Material

Since prehistoric times, mankind has recognised the role of iron in health care and therapy. While discussing iron-based metallurgical artifacts, the term "steel" is more preferred over the word "iron," which is generally used to refer to the pure element Fe. According to the ancient Indian Vedic scriptures and Roman history, Fe has been used in medical materials for prosthetics during the periods of 1200 BC and 200 BC (Flood 1996; Marin et al. 2020). Even though the language is not unambiguous in its interpretation, the allusion to the usage of iron qualifies as the first reference to the concept of a limb prosthetic. The approximate time period corresponds to the early emergence and spread of iron smelting in those regions (Tewari 2003). Iron was probably chosen as a symbol and is related to the superior characteristics of what was a comparatively recent discovery at the time: a bulk iron prosthesis

VP. Md. Rabeeh and T. Hanas, *Biodegradable Iron Implants: Development, Processing, and Applications*, SpringerBriefs in Materials,
https://doi.org/10.1007/978-3-031-82099-1_2

implant would have been too heavy to wear satisfactorily. In 200 AD, iron was used as a dental implant, as evidenced by the discovery of a cadaver in the Gallo-Roman mausoleum of Chantambre (Crubezy et al. 1998). With the invention of stainless steel in the early nineteenth century, it was used as a temporary implant for therapeutic purposes. Such implants were removed by a second surgery once the tissue was healed. However, iron as a degradable implant material was not investigated until 2001. Peuster et al. (2001) published the first research on the effects of the implantation of a degradable Fe-based cardiovascular stent in New Zealand white rabbits. The implant showed a very little inflammatory response and exhibited low thrombogenesis. Later, because of the exceptional features of Fe, a series of experiments were undertaken by Hermawan et al. (2008, 2013) and other several research groups to tailor the degrading behaviour of Fe and Fe-based materials (Liu and Zheng 2011; Hufenbach et al. 2017; Mostavan et al. 2017; Sharipova et al. 2019). However, there are no products available in the global market developed from Fe that can be effectively used as degradable metallic implants. The main challenge for developing such a material is the very slow degradation rate of Fe in the physiological environment. Scientists are working on strategies to accelerate the degradation rate of iron-based compounds in the human body in order to make them more biodegradable for use in temporary implant applications. New possible compositions and manufacturing techniques are being tried to tailor the rate of degradation while maintaining the mechanical integrity. Elements such as Mn, Pd, Si, Ag, and rare earth elements are incorporated with Fe in order to achieve a controlled degradation rate (Rabeeh and Hanas 2022). Compounds such as HA and iron-bio ceramic are also being added to ferrous materials to improve their mechanical properties, degradation rate, bioactivity, and biocompatibility. Several manufacturing techniques are also employed to generate a diverse range of biodegradable iron-based materials, including vacuum induction melting, molecular beam epitaxy, spark plasma sintering, melting furnaces, powder metallurgy, electroforming, and equal channel angular pressing (Gorejová et al. 2019). Figure 2.1 shows the statistics of the publications year-wise and region-wise. However, there are no products available in the global market developed from Fe that can be effectively used as degradable metallic implants.

2.3   Fe in Human Body

Iron is an essential element for the human body for the production of haemoglobin and is a vital element involved in human physiological activities. It is a cofactor for a large number of enzymes and proteins involved in a wide range of biological activities such as oxygen binding, DNA synthesis, and redox enzymatic activity (Mueller et al. 2006; Zhu et al. 2009a, b). In addition, Fe is also involved in many other activities, such as the transport of electrons inside cells, the reduction of ribonucleotides and dinitrogen, and the storage as well as the release of molecular oxygen. As it is involved in a wide variety of biological processes and is directly controlled by the human body, either a surplus or a shortage can be detrimental (Papanikolaou and Pantopoulos

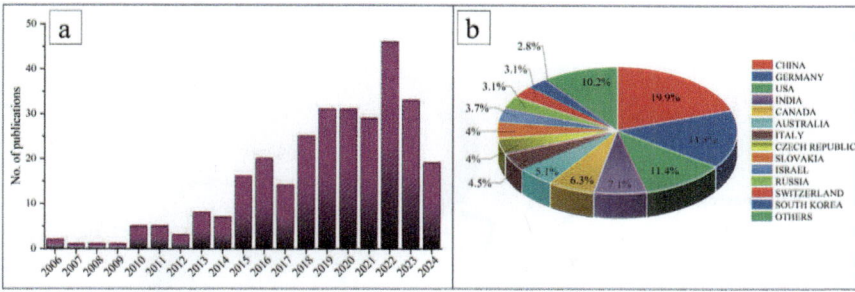

Fig. 2.1 Recent research on Fe-based degradable implants (keywords: Iron; biodegradable; implants); **a** Year-wise statistics and **b** Region-wise statistics. *Source* Web of science, 10th Oct 2024

2005). Figure 2.2 shows the dynamic distribution of Fe in the human body. For adults, the average oral consumption of iron is 10–20 mg/day, and approximately 10% of this is extracted by the digestive tract. The highest permissible intake of iron is limited to 45 mg/day in adults (Seiler and Sigel 1988; Trumbo et al. 2001). The majority of iron consumed is used to produce haemoglobin and it is stored as ferritin and haemosiderin in various organs such as the liver, spleen, bone marrow, duodenum, and muscle tissues (Abbaspour et al. 2014; Saito 2014). Nevertheless, iron is considered one of the best biocompatible metals, which does not harm tissues in the physiological environment (Papanikolaou and Pantopoulos 2005).

2.4 Degradation Process of Fe in Physiological Environment

In the physiological environment, the degradation of Fe takes place through electrochemical reactions, (2.1), (2.2) and (2.3) (Zheng et al. 2014, 2017).

$$Fe \rightarrow Fe^{2+} + 2e^- \text{(anodic reaction)} \qquad (2.1)$$

$$O_2 + 2H_2O + 4e^- \rightarrow 4OH^- \text{(cathodic reaction)} \qquad (2.2)$$

In aqueous media, this Fe^{2+} and OH^- will form ferrous hydroxide:

$$Fe^{2+} + 2OH^- \rightarrow Fe(OH)_2 \downarrow \qquad (2.3)$$

Due to the alkalization of the solution and presence of oxygen in the physiological fluid, some ferrous hydroxide transforms into ferric hydroxide as shown by (2.4) and (2.5).

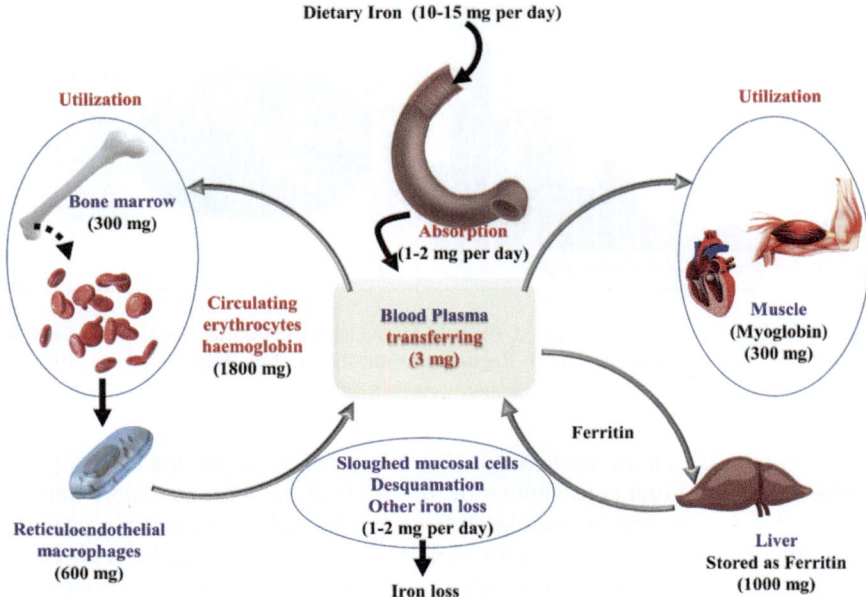

Fig. 2.2 Dynamic distribution of iron in the human body (Reprinted with permission of Springer Nature from Rabeeh and Hanas 2022)

$$4Fe(OH)_2 + O_2 + 2H_2O \rightarrow 4Fe(OH)_3 \downarrow \qquad (2.4)$$

$$Fe(OH)_2 + 2FeO(OH)+ \rightarrow Fe_3O_4 \downarrow +H_2O \qquad (2.5)$$

Figure 2.3 presents a schematic representation of the degradation mechanism of Fe-based biodegradable materials in the physiological environment. As illustrated in Fig. 2.3a, reactions (2.1) to (2.5) occur spontaneously at locations where galvanic coupling is present. Metallic iron undergoes immediate oxidation upon exposure to bodily fluids due to the anodic reaction (2.1), with the released electrons driving the cathodic reduction of dissolved oxygen. Figure 2.3b demonstrates that this process is accompanied by the adsorption of organic molecules such as lipids, proteins, and amino acids, along with the formation of degradation products through reactions (2.3)–(2.5). Given the high concentrations of inorganic ions like Cl⁻ in body fluids, the protective hydroxide layer on the iron surface breaks down continuously, promoting ongoing degradation (Paramitha et al. 2016). In addition to the corrosion product layer, cells adhere to the surface, proliferating to form tissue. Occasionally, irregular degradation fragments detach from the surface and are removed from the site, as depicted in Fig. 2.3d.

The formation of calcium phosphate (apatite), along with hydroxide and oxide layers on the surface of Fe, contributes to reducing its degradation rate in the early

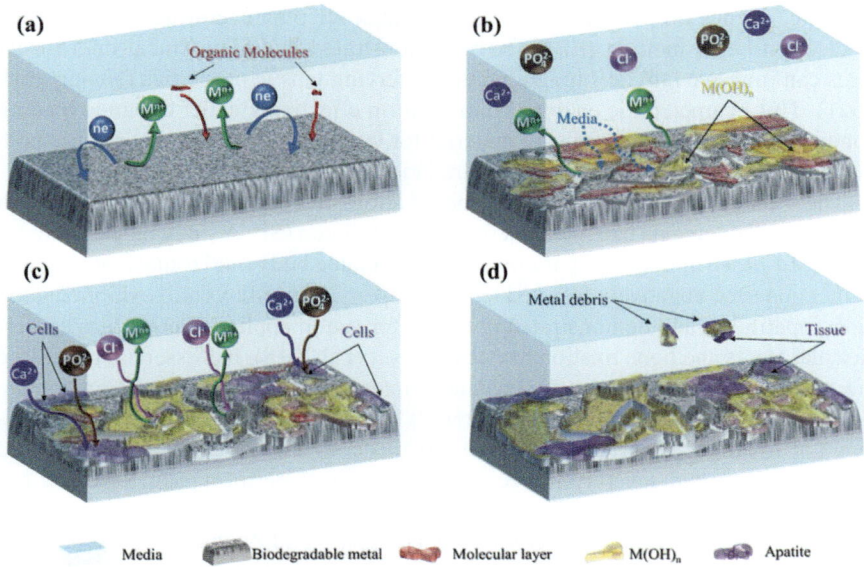

Fig. 2.3 Degradation mechanism of Fe-based BMs (Reprinted with permission of Springer Nature from Rabeeh and Hanas 2022)

stages of dynamic immersion (Zhu et al. 2009a, b). However, concerns over the persistence of degradation layers in vivo appear unfounded. Studies by Moravej et al. (2010) and Wegener et al. (2021) have shown that degradation products are effectively removed by macrophages, with no adverse effects resulting from local accumulation. Furthermore, the degradation products of Fe show no significant toxicity to human tissues. Excess Fe ions are readily transported through body fluids and efficiently excreted via sloughed mucosal cells, sweat, and desquamation of skin and hair (Peuster et al. 2001; Ulum et al. 2014; Scarcello and Lison 2020).

2.5 Mechanical Properties of Degradable Fe

Fe exhibits promising mechanical properties that make it a suitable candidate for orthopedic implant applications. Its high yield strength, elastic modulus, and ductility are particularly advantageous for load-bearing implants, where the material is expected to withstand mechanical load during the healing process. The mechanical properties of pure Fe include a tensile strength of approximately 370 MPa and an elastic modulus of about 200 GPa, which are adequate for some applications but often insufficient for more demanding orthopaedic uses (Hermawan et al. 2010a). Recent research has underscored the importance of tailoring the mechanical properties of Fe-based alloys to meet the specific requirements of orthopedic applications. For example, studies on pure iron produced via additive manufacturing methods such as electron beam melting (EBM) have demonstrated that hierarchical microstructures can improve fatigue strength while preserving tensile properties (Huang et al. 2021). This characteristic enables Fe to perform effectively under dynamic loading conditions, making it a promising material for temporary implants that require both mechanical strength and controlled degradation.

The mechanical performance of Fe-based alloys can be further enhanced through alloying with elements like manganese (Mn) and silicon (Si). A study on the behavior of Fe–Mn-based alloys during immersion in simulated body fluid found that although immersion time negatively affected tensile properties, the alloys still exhibited good biocompatibility and demonstrated potential for use in applications such as cardiovascular stents and bone fixation devices (Drevet et al 2018). It is essential to achieve the required balance between mechanical integrity and safe degradation for the successful implementation of these materials in medical settings. However, the challenge of hydrogen embrittlement (HE) remains a significant concern for Fe-based materials, as it can severely impact their mechanical performance. Research has shown that the presence of hydrogen can lead to substantial degradation in mechanical properties, particularly under tensile loading (Xu and Zhang 2017). Addressing this issue through advanced material design and processing techniques will be critical to improve the reliability of degradable iron implants. Continued exploration of these areas will drive innovation in implant technology and contribute to improved patient outcomes in orthopedic and other medical applications.

Table: Summary of mechanical properties of biodegradable iron-based implant materials.

Material	Tensile Strength (MPa)	Yield Strength (MPa)	Elongation (%)	Young's Modulus (GPa)	References
Pure Iron	370	200	20	210	Hermawan et al. (2010a, b)
Fe-35Mn Alloy	450	210	15	35	(Hermawan et al. 2007)
Fe-30Mn Alloy	~400	~200	~15	~40	Zheng et al. (2014)
Fe-Cu Alloy	~350	~180	~20	~200	(Gorejová et al. 2019)
Fe–Mn–Cu Alloy	~450	~230	~15	~40	Zhang et al. (2024)
Fe–Mn–Si Alloy	~420	~210	~18	~45	Zheng et al. (2014)
Fe–Ni–Mn Alloy	~500	~220	~14	~38	Zhang et al. (2024)
Fe-W	–	180–300	–	–	Cheng and Zheng (2013)

(continued)

(continued)

Material	Tensile Strength (MPa)	Yield Strength (MPa)	Elongation (%)	Young's Modulus (GPa)	References
Fe-CNT	–	200–300	–	–	Cheng and Zheng (2013)
Fe-2Pd	–	127.2	–	–	Čapek et al. (2016)
Fe-2Ag	–	116.2	–	–	Čapek et al. (2016)
Fe-2C	–	113.3	–	–	Čapek et al. (2016)
Fe-HA	–	325	–	–	Ulum et al. (2014)
Fe-BCP	–	312	–	–	Ulum et al. (2014)
Fe-TCP	–	312	–	–	Ulum et al. (2014)
Fe/Mg$_2$Si	–	290–500	–	–	Sikora-Jasinska et al. (2017)
Fe-(20–35)Mn	–	230–440	–	–	Heiden et al. (2015)
Porous Fe-30Mn	–	48.2	–	–	Dehestani et al. (2017)
Fe-30Mn	–	134..2	–	–	Dehestani et al. (2017)
Fe-30Mn-6Si	–	177.8	–	–	Čapek et al. (2016)
Fe-2Pd	–	279.4	–	–	Čapek et al. (2017)
Fe	–	73	–	–	Čapek et al. (2017)
Fe-2Pd	–	845..8	–	–	Čapek et al. (2017)
Fe-2Pd (Porous)	–	14.7	–	–	Čapek et al. (2017)
Fe–Mn	–	189	–	–	Hong et al. (2016)
Fe-30Mn	–	106	–	–	Liu and Zheng (2011)
Fe-30Mn-1C	–	373	-	–	Hufenbach et al. (2017)

2.6 Advantages and Limitations of Fe for Implants

Fe is known for its versatility and mechanical properties. Unlike biodegradable polymers that are used to make the vast majority of degradable implants, metals like Fe offer superior strength, which makes them the ideal choice for load-bearing applications. The performance of the majority of those clinical devices made of biodegradable metals in demanding stress environments is likely to depend on the physiological state of the implanted site. The implant is expected to withstand not only the harsh environment but also the mechanical loads, such as tension, compression, fatigue and shear stresses. (Zheng et al. 2014). Fe and Fe-based alloys have gained significant importance due to their excellent mechanical properties and biocompatibility (Hermawan et al. 2007, 2010b). Moreover, the degradation of Fe-based alloys is not accompanied by hydrogen evolution that hinders blood flow, as in the case of Mg (Li et al. 2018).

The major advantages of Fe-based alloys can be listed as follows:

- Excellent load-bearing properties such as high strength and toughness.
- A high machinability index, as well as dimensional stability which are critical when designing complicated geometric shapes for orthopaedic use.
- Fe is biocompatible and biodegradable.
- Degradation products or by-products are not harmful to the human body.
- As an important cation for human metabolism, Fe serves as a cofactor for numerous enzymes, including those involved in haemoglobin formation.

The primary limitation of using iron for temporary orthopedic implants lies in its relatively slow degradation rate within the human body. The ideal timeframe for a biodegradable metallic implant is between 6 and 18 months (Prakasam et al. 2017). If the implant remains beyond this period, it may lead to complications such as long-term endothelial dysfunction, delayed re-endothelialization, thrombogenicity, stress shielding, and other persistent local responses (Wegener et al. 2020). The elastic modulus of iron is significantly higher than that of bone tissue and can result in stress shielding, which reduces the stimulus for new bone growth and impacts bone remodelling causing a decrease in bone density (Nagels et al. 2003; Niinomi et al. 2012).

While iron degradation does not typically produce harmful by-products, some in vitro studies on Fe-containing stents have shown the accumulation of insoluble degradation products (IDPs) near the implantation site, potentially damaging surrounding tissues (Fagali et al. 2020). The redox chemistry of iron also poses certain risks, primarily related to Fenton chemistry. Iron exists mainly in two oxidation states, ferrous (Fe^{2+}) and ferric (Fe^{3+}). In aerobic conditions, molecular oxygen accelerates the conversion of ferrous iron to its more stable ferric form (Lesjak and Srai 2019). Ferrous iron (Fe^{2+}) can generate superoxide anions, which may subsequently produce hydrogen peroxide (H_2O_2). Through the Fenton reaction, this H_2O_2 reacts with Fe^{2+} to form highly reactive hydroxyl radicals ($HO\cdot$), which can be harmful to proteins and nearby tissues.

Table 2.1 Summaty of benefits and limitations of Fe-based systems as degradable implant

Benefits of Fe-based system	Limitations of Fe-based system
Biocompatibility and Biodegradability: Exhibit favorable interactions with biological tissues, making them suitable for medical applications. They degrade in physiological environments, reducing the risk of long-term foreign body reactions	**Slow Degradation Rate**: The slow degradation of Fe may limit its effectiveness in applications requiring rapid resorption
Mechanical Strength and Toughness: Offers superior strength and toughness, making it suitable for load-bearing orthopedic implants	**High Elastic Modulus:** The high elastic modulus of Fe compared to natural bone can lead to stress shielding effects
Essential Nutrient: Iron is vital for metabolism and is a co-factor for many enzymes, including those involved in hemoglobin synthesis	**Insoluble Degradation Products (IDP):** Risk of insoluble products forming at the implant site may harm surrounding tissues
Rarity of Hyper-Iron Cases: Instances of hyper-iron conditions are uncommon, suggesting low risk from iron-based implants	**Potential Toxicity Concerns:** Long-term effects of iron accumulation in tissues need further investigation for safety
Machinability and Dimensional Stability: Good machinability and stability are essential for creating complex implants	

These challenges have prompted extensive research over the past two decades aimed at accelerating the degradation of biodegradable Fe-based materials while minimizing the accumulation of IDPs. Furthermore, efforts have been made to modify their mechanical properties to meet clinical requirements, allowing for optimal bone integration, healing, and degradation without significant stress shielding. The key benefits and limitations of Fe-based systems are summarized given in Table 2.1.

2.7 Validation of Degradable Fe

To ensure the clinical viability, any degradable metallic implants must undergo rigorous validation through both preclinical and clinical studies. The primary aim of these studies is to confirm the material's degradability, biocompatibility, and effectiveness in supporting tissue healing while avoiding long-term adverse effects. This process encompasses in vitro (laboratory-based) evaluations, in vivo (animal-based) studies, and potential future clinical trials in humans.

2.7.1 In Vitro Studies and Material Properties

The validation process for Fe-based biodegradable implants begins with a thorough in vitro investigation on the performance. Several studies have examined the degradation behaviour of Fe in simulated physiological environments, such as simulated body fluid (SBF), Hank's balanced salt solution (HBSS) and phosphate-buffered saline (PBS), which mimic the conditions inside the human body. These studies consistently show that Fe degrades at a relatively slow rate compared to other biodegradable metals like Mg or Zn.

In vitro studies also reports the release of iron corrosion products, primarily iron oxide (FeO) and iron hydroxide ($Fe(OH)_2$). These products have been demonstrated to be relatively non-toxic, but concerns remain about their accumulation over time, especially if the rate of degradation is too slow to allow complete absorption of the implant within a clinically relevant timeframe (Peuster et al. 2001). The studies also revealed that mechanical properties of iron, such as its tensile strength and ductility, are favourable for load-bearing applications, as they are close to those of stainless steel, but with the added benefit of being biodegradable.

In vitro biocompatibility studies are essential for evaluating the suitability of biodegradable metals for medical implants. These studies assess how these materials interact with biological systems, focusing on their effects on cell viability, metabolic activity, and overall biocompatibility. Although in vitro studies do not fully replicate the complex environment of living tissues in contact with implant materials, they serve as an essential preliminary step in evaluating biocompatibility when appropriate models are employed. To mimic the effects of release of Fe ion, researchers introduced Fe^{3+} solutions into cell culture media, enabling the study of its impact on cell viability. This approach revealed a notable reduction in mitochondrial activity at Fe^{3+} concentrations exceeding 2 mM, as well as increased lipid peroxidation in CHO–K1 cells. On the other hand, iron solutions incubated for 1 to 3 days with endothelial cells showed no toxicity at concentrations below 50 mg/mL (Fagali et al. 2015).

The degradation products of iron from medical devices are typically analyzed using direct or indirect contact tests in accordance with ISO 10993–5 standards. These guidelines define the conditions for extracting released products (such as cm^2 or mg of sample per mL of extractant), conducting cytotoxicity tests, and selecting appropriate cell lines. Commonly used cell lines are often derived from rodents, including L929 fibroblast, BALB/3T3 fibroblasts, J774A.1 macrophages, and CHO–K1 epithelial cells, which are suited for toxicology assessments but may not accurately represent the tissues surrounding implant. Only a limited number of studies have investigated more relevant human models, such as human endothelial cells (HUV-EC-C), smooth muscle cells (SMCs), adipose tissue-derived stem cells (ADSCs) and osteosarcoma cells (MG-63) (Fagali et al. 2020).

Cytotoxicity assessments of iron corrosion products are typically conducted by placing iron samples in a physiological buffer or culture medium, with the released products later introduced to the cells for testing. Schematic representation of in vitro tests for the biocompatibility evaluation is given in Fig. 2.4. Another technique involves using culture inserts with permeable polymeric membranes (such as polyethylene terephthalate, polyvinylidene difluoride, or nitrocellulose), allowing soluble compounds to diffuse. Cell viability is then assessed after 24 to 72 h, usually through metabolic activity tests like MTT Assay and Alamar blue. Other parameters such as cell morphology, reactive oxygen species (ROS) production, gene expression, and cell proliferation are also examined. There is broad agreement that soluble iron degradation products are not toxic to various cell types, including fibroblasts, CHO–K1 cells, human endothelial cells, smooth muscle cells, and adipose-derived stem cells (ADSCs).

Most in vitro evaluations occur in static conditions, causing Fe ions and ROS to accumulate at levels higher than in vivo, where blood flow disperses them. To better mimic in vivo conditions, dynamic systems like bioreactors, with circulating medium, are used to assess cytotoxicity and corrosion. Ex vivo studies simulate blood flow to account for shear stress and material degradation, using mock vessels or arteries. Such studies reported that physiological flow increases iron degradation compared to static conditions (Huang et al. 2014). These findings underscore the promising role of iron-based materials in promoting cellular responses critical for successful integration and functionality in bone tissue engineering.

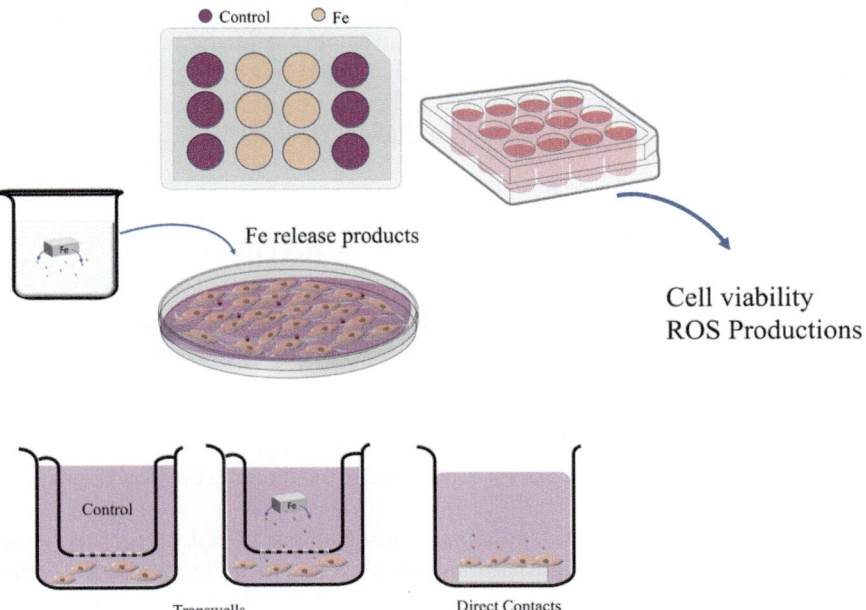

Fig. 2.4 Schematic representation of in vitro tests for the biocompatibility evaluation of Fe samples (MTT test of ADSCs for indirect contact evaluation of iron released products)

2.7.2 *In Vivo Studies and Biocompatibility*

In vivo studies are critical for assessing the biological behaviour of iron-based implants in a living organism. Several animal studies have been conducted to evaluate the degradation, tissue response, and safety of Fe-based implants. Peuster et al. (2006) performed one of the pioneering studies on iron stents in a pig model. They found that iron stents showed good mechanical stability and no acute toxicity or excessive inflammatory response in the short term. However, long-term follow-up revealed that the degradation of iron was significantly slower than anticipated. After 18 months, a considerable portion of the iron stent remained, indicating that the material had not degraded at a rate compatible with the expected healing of vascular tissue. In a study involving rabbit models, Hermawan et al. (2010a) investigated the performance of pure iron implants in bone. The results showed minimal inflammatory response and good biocompatibility, but again highlighted the slow degradation of the material. Bone healing around the iron implants was observed, with the implant maintaining its mechanical integrity for a prolonged period. While this could be beneficial in applications requiring long-term support, the eventual need for faster degradation to match bone remodelling remains a significant challenge.

Additionally, iron-based materials have shown a relatively benign tissue response in terms of macrophage activity and inflammatory cytokine release. Studies have found that iron degradation products do not elicit severe immune responses, unlike some other metals such as cobalt or nickel. This makes iron a promising candidate in terms of long-term biocompatibility. However, slow degradation raises concerns about iron ion accumulation in tissues, which could potentially lead to localized iron overload and subsequent pathologies, though no conclusive evidence of such outcomes has been reported in short-term studies (Zhang et al. 2010).

2.7.3 *Clinical Implications and Future Directions*

While clinical data on Fe-based biodegradable implants in humans are still lacking, the in vitro and in vivo results from animal studies provide a promising foundation for future clinical trials. The key challenge remains optimizing the degradation rate of iron-based implants to match the biological healing process, particularly in bone and cardiovascular applications. Innovations such as alloying, surface coatings, and the development of porous structures show potential in overcoming the slow degradation hurdle.

It is also important to consider the long-term systemic effects of iron ion release and accumulation. While short-term studies have not identified any major safety concerns, the potential for localized iron overload in tissues must be addressed through extended follow-up studies and clinical trials. Moreover, the ability of the body to metabolize and clear iron ions effectively should be evaluated to ensure that no long-term toxicities arise from iron-based degradable implants.

References

Abbaspour N, Hurrell R, Kelishadi R (2014) Review on iron and its importance for human health. J Res Med Sci 19:164–174

Čapek J, Stehlíková K, Michalcová A, Msallamová S, Vojtěch D (2016) Microstructure mechanical and corrosion properties of biodegradable powder metallurgical Fe-2 wt% X (X = Pd Ag and C) alloys Materials Chemistry and Physics 181501–511. https://doi.org/10.1016/j.matchemphys.2016.06.087

Čapek J, Msallamová Š, Jablonská E, Lipov J, Vojtěch D (2017) A novel high-strength and highly corrosive biodegradable Fe–Pd alloy: Structural, mechanical and in vitro corrosion and cytotoxicity study. Mater Sci Eng C 79:550–562. https://doi.org/10.1016/j.msec.2017.05.100

Cheng J, Zheng YF (2013) In vitro study on newly designed biodegradable Fe-X composites (X = W, CNT) prepared by spark plasma sintering. J Biomed Mater Res—Part B Appl Biomater 101:485–497. https://doi.org/10.1002/jbm.b.32783

Crubezy E, Murail P, Girard L, Bernadou JP (1998) False teeth of the Roman world. Nature 391:29. https://doi.org/10.1038/34067

Dehestani M, Trumble K, Wang H, Stanciu L A (2017) Effects of microstructure and heat treatment on mechanical properties and corrosion behavior of powder metallurgy derived Fe–30Mn alloy. Mater Sci Eng A 703:214–226. https://doi.org/10.1016/j.msea.2017.07.054

Drevet R, Zhukova Y, Malikova P et al (2018) Martensitic transformations and mechanical and corrosion properties of Fe–Mn–Si alloys for biodegradable medical implants. Metall Mater Trans A Phys Metall Mater Sci 49:1006–1013. https://doi.org/10.1007/s11661-017-4458-2

John E (2011) Nature's building blocks an A–Z guide to the elements, 2nd edn. Oxford University Press

Fagali NS, Grillo CA, Puntarulo S, Lorenzo F, de Mele MA (2015) Cytotoxicity of corrosion products of degradable Fe-based stents: relevance of pH and insoluble products. Colloids Surf B Biointerfaces 128:480–488. https://doi.org/10.1016/j.colsurfb.2015.02.047

Fagali NS, Madrid MA, Pérez MacEda BT et al (2020) Effect of degradation products of iron-bioresorbable implants on the physiological behavior of macrophages in vitro. Metallomics 12:1841–1850. https://doi.org/10.1039/D0MT00151A

Flood GD (1996) An introduction to Hinduism. Cambridge University Press

Gorejová R, Haverová L, Oriňaková R et al (2019) Recent advancements in Fe-based biodegradable materials for bone repair. J Mater Sci 54:1913–1947. https://doi.org/10.1007/s10853-018-3011-z

Heiden M, Walker E, Nauman E, Stanciu L (2015) Evolution of novel bioresorbable iron-manganese implant surfaces and their degradation behaviors in vitro. J Biomed Mater Res Part A 103:185–193. https://doi.org/10.1002/jbm.a.35155

Hermawan H, Alamdari H, Mantovani D, Dubé D (2008) Iron–manganese: new class of metallic degradable biomaterials prepared by powder metallurgy. Powder Metall 51:38–45. https://doi.org/10.1179/174329008X284868

Hermawan H, Dubé D, Mantovani D (2010a) Degradable metallic biomaterials for cardiovascular applications. In: Metals for biomedical devices. Elsevier Ltd, pp 379–404

Hermawan H, Dubé D, Mantovani D (2007) Development of degradable Fe-35Mn alloy for biomedical application. Adv Mat Res 15–17:107–112. https://doi.org/10.4028/www.scientific.net/AMR.15-17.107

Hermawan H, Dubé D, Mantovani D (2010b) Degradable metallic biomaterials: Design and development of Fe–Mn alloys for stents. J Biomed Mater Res A 93:1–11. https://doi.org/10.1002/jbm.a.32224

Hermawan H, Mantovani D (2013) Process of prototyping coronary stents from biodegradable Fe-Mn alloys. Acta Biomater 9:8585–8592. https://doi.org/10.1016/j.actbio.2013.04.027

Hong D, Chou DT, Velikokhatnyi OI, Roy A, Lee B, Swink I, Issaev I, Kuhn HA, Kumta PN (2016) Binder-jetting 3D printing and alloy development of new biodegradable Fe-Mn-Ca/Mg alloys. Acta Biomater 45:375–386. https://doi.org/10.1016/j.actbio.2016.08.032

Huang CC, Lam TN, Amalia L et al (2021) Tailoring grain sizes of the biodegradable iron-based alloys by pre-additive manufacturing microalloying. Sci Rep 11. https://doi.org/10.1038/S41 598-021-89022-9

Huang T, Cheng J, Zheng YF (2014) In vitro degradation and biocompatibility of Fe–Pd and Fe–Pt composites fabricated by spark plasma sintering. Mater Sci Eng C 35:43–53. https://doi.org/10. 1016/j.msec.2013.10.023

Hufenbach J, Wendrock H, Kochta F et al (2017) Novel biodegradable Fe–Mn–C–S alloy with superior mechanical and corrosion properties. Mater Lett 186:330–333. https://doi.org/10.1016/ j.matlet.2016.10.037

ISO 10993–5:2009—Biological evaluation of medical devices—Part 5: Tests for in vitro cytotoxi-city

Lesjak M, Srai SKS (2019) Role of dietary flavonoids in iron homeostasis. Pharmaceuticals 12:119. https://doi.org/10.3390/PH12030119

Li Y, Jahr H, Lietaert K et al (2018) Additively manufactured biodegradable porous iron. Acta Biomater 77:380–393. https://doi.org/10.1016/j.actbio.2018.07.011

Liu B, Zheng YF (2011) Effects of alloying elements (Mn Co, Al, W, Sn, B, C and S) on biodegrad-ability and in vitro biocompatibility of pure iron. Acta Biomater 7:1407–1420. https://doi.org/ 10.1016/J.ACTBIO.2010.11.001

Marin E, Boschetto F, Pezzotti G (2020) Biomaterials and biocompatibility: an historical overview. J Biomed Mater Res A 108:1617–1633. https://doi.org/10.1002/JBM.A.36930

Moravej M, Purnama A, Fiset M et al (2010) Electroformed pure iron as a new biomaterial for degradable stents: In vitro degradation and preliminary cell viability studies. Acta Biomater 6:1843–1851. https://doi.org/10.1016/j.actbio.2010.01.008

Mostavan A, Paternoster C, Tolouei R et al (2017) Effect of electrolyte composition and deposition current for Fe/Fe-P electroformed bilayers for biodegradable metallic medical applications. Mater Sci Eng C 70:195–206. https://doi.org/10.1016/j.msec.2016.08.026

Mueller PP, May T, Perz A et al (2006) Control of smooth muscle cell proliferation by ferrous iron. Biomaterials 27:2193–2200. https://doi.org/10.1016/j.biomaterials.2005.10.042

Nagels J, Stokdijk M, Rozing PM (2003) Stress shielding and bone resorption in shoulder arthroplasty. J Shoulder Elbow Surg 12:35–39. https://doi.org/10.1067/mse.2003.22

Niinomi M, Nakai M, Hieda J (2012) Development of new metallic alloys for biomedical applications. Acta Biomater 8:3888–3903. https://doi.org/10.1016/j.actbio.2012.06.037

Papanikolaou G, Pantopoulos K (2005) Iron metabolism and toxicity. Toxicol Appl Pharmacol 202:199–211

Prakasam M, Locs J, Salma-Ancane K, Loca D, Largeteau A, Berzina-Cimdina L (2017) Biodegrad-able materials and metallic implants—a review. J Funct Biomater 8:44. https://doi.org/10.3390/ jfb8040044

Paramitha D, Ulum MF, Purnama A, et al (2016) Monitoring degradation products and metal ions in vivo. In: Monitoring and evaluation of biomaterials and their performance in vivo. Elsevier Ltd, pp 19–44

Peuster M, Hesse C, Schloo T, Fink C, Beerbaum P, von Schnakenburg C (2006) Long-term biocom-patibility of a corrodible peripheral iron stent in the porcine descending aorta. Biomaterials 27:4955–4962. https://doi.org/10.1016/j.msec.2013.10.023

Peuster M, Wohlsein P, Brügmann M et al (2001) A novel approach to temporary stenting : degradable cardiovascular stents produced from corrodible metal—results 6–18 months after implantation into New Zealand white rabbits. Heart 1000:563–569

Rabeeh VPM, Hanas T (2022) Enhancing biointerfacial properties of porous pure iron by gold sputtering for degradable implant applications. Mater Today Commun 31:103492. https://doi. org/10.1016/J.MTCOMM.2022.103492

Saito H (2014) Metabolism of iron stores. Nagoya J Med Sci 76:235–254

Scarcello E, Lison D (2020) Are Fe-based stenting materials biocompatible? A critical review of in vitro and in vivo studies. J Funct Biomater 11:2

Seiler HG, Sigel H (1988) Handbook on toxicity of inorganic compounds. Marcel Dekker, United States

Sharipova A, Gotman I, Psakhie SG, Gutmanas EY (2019) Biodegradable nanocomposite Fe–Ag load-bearing scaffolds for bone healing. J Mech Behav Biomed Mater 98:246–254. https://doi.org/10.1016/j.jmbbm.2019.06.033

Sikora-Jasinska M, Paternoster C, Mostaed E, Tolouei R, Casati, R, Vedani M, Mantovani D (2017) Synthesis, mechanical properties and corrosion behavior of powder metallurgy processed Fe/Mg^2Si composites for biodegradable implant applications. Mater Sci Eng C 81:511–521. https://doi.org/10.1016/j.msec.2017.07.049

Tewari R (2003) The origins of iron working in India: new evidence from the Central Ganga Plain and the Eastern Vindhyas. Antiquity 77:536–544. https://doi.org/10.1017/S0003598X00092590

Trumbo P, Yates AA, Schlicker S, Poos M (2001) Dietary reference intakes: vitamin A, vitamin K, arsenic, boron, chromium, copper, iodine, iron, manganese, molybdenum, nickel, silicon, vanadium, and zinc. J Am Diet Assoc 101:294–301. https://doi.org/10.1016/S0002-8223(01)00078-5

Ulum MF, Arafat A, Noviana D et al (2014) In vitro and in vivo degradation evaluation of novel iron-bioceramic composites for bone implant applications. Mater Sci Eng C 36:336–344. https://doi.org/10.1016/j.msec.2013.12.022

Wegener B, Behnke M, Milz S, et al (2021) Local and systemic inflammation after implantation of a novel iron based porous degradable bone replacement material in sheep model. Scientific Reports 11:1 11:1–11. https://doi.org/10.1038/s41598-021-91296-y

Wegener B, Sichler A, Milz S et al (2020) Development of a novel biodegradable porous iron-based implant for bone replacement. Sci Rep 10:1–10. https://doi.org/10.1038/s41598-020-66289-y

Xu Q, Zhang J (2017) Novel methods for prevention of hydrogen embrittlement in iron. Sci Rep 7:16927. https://doi.org/10.1038/s41598-017-17263-8

Zhang E, Chen H, Shen F (2010) Biocorrosion properties and blood and cell compatibility of pure iron as a biodegradable biomaterial. J Mater Sci Mater Med 21:2151–2163. https://doi.org/10.1007/s10856-010-4070-0

Zhang Y, Roux C, Rouchaud A, Meddahi-Pellé A, Gueguen V, Mangeney C, Sun F, Pavon-Djavid G, Luo Y (2024) Recent advances in Fe-based bioresorbable stents: materials design and biosafety. Bioact Mater 31:333–354. https://doi.org/10.1016/j.bioactmat.2023.07.024

Zheng Y, Xu X, Xu Z et al (2017) Development of Fe-based degradable metallic biomaterials. In: Metallic biomaterials. Wiley-VCH Verlag GmbH & Co. KGaA, pp 113–160

Zheng YF, Gu XN, Witte F (2014) Biodegradable metals. Mater Sci Eng R Rep 77:1–34

Zhu S, Huang N, Shu H et al (2009a) Corrosion resistance and blood compatibility of lanthanum ion implanted pure iron by MEVVA. Appl Surf Sci 256:99–104. https://doi.org/10.1016/j.apsusc.2009.07.082

Zhu S, Huang N, Xu L et al (2009b) Biocompatibility of pure iron: In vitro assessment of degradation kinetics and cytotoxicity on endothelial cells. Mater Sci Eng, C 29:1589–1592. https://doi.org/10.1016/J.MSEC.2008.12.019

Chapter 3
Biodegradable Fe: Materials Development

3.1 Overview

A range of manufacturing and processing techniques are employed to enhance the degradation rate, optimize biological responses, and fine-tune the mechanical properties of iron (Fe) for use in degradable implant applications. These methods are crucial for addressing the inherent challenges associated with Fe-based materials, such as their slow degradation rates and need for biocompatibility. Researchers have placed significant focus on the selection of appropriate manufacturing routes and processing methods to achieve Fe-based materials with the desired degradation profiles and mechanical characteristics suited for biomedical use. This chapter focuses specifically on the various manufacturing techniques used to produce Fe-based biodegradable metals, highlighting the approaches that can modulate their degradation behaviour to meet the requirements of temporary implant applications.

3.2 Manufacturing of Fe-Based Biodegradable Metal

The fabrication methods used to develop Fe-based biodegradable metallic materials can be broadly categorized as powder metallurgy, casting, electrodeposition, additive manufacturing, and other techniques as illustrated in Fig. 3.1. Each of these methods presents unique advantages and limitations when applied to the production of Fe-based biodegradable devices.

© The Author(s), under exclusive license to Springer Nature Switzerland AG 2025
VP. Md. Rabeeh and T. Hanas, *Biodegradable Iron Implants: Development, Processing, and Applications*, SpringerBriefs in Materials,
https://doi.org/10.1007/978-3-031-82099-1_3

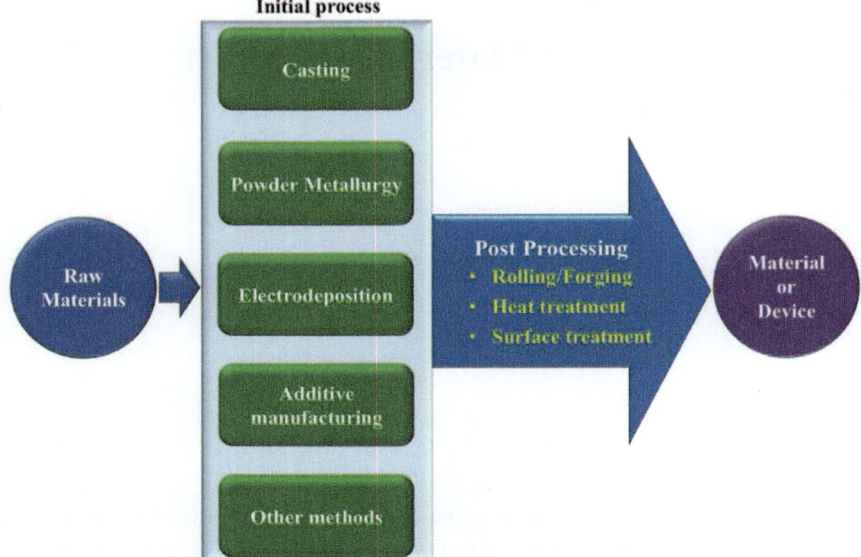

Fig. 3.1 Manufacturing methods for Fe-based BMs

3.3 Powder Metallurgy

The powder metallurgy (PM) route is a prominent technique for developing Fe-based BMs due to its versatility in controlling material properties and microstructure (Hermawan et al. 2008, 2010b; Cheng and Zheng 2013; Zheng et al. 2014; Oriňaková et al. 2016). In this process, fine iron powders are mixed with alloying elements and compacted into the desired shape prior to sintering, a high-temperature treatment below the melting point of iron. The inherent versatility of PM allows to produce complex components with tailored geometries and specific features, starting from metal powders. This process offers significant advantages, including the ability to control microstructural features such as porosity, and grain size as well as the mechanical properties. A proper selection of powder composition, compaction techniques, and sintering conditions can help in achieving the desired performance, making it a preferred method for developing biodegradable metal implants. Various powder metallurgical methods used for making Fe based degradable materials are shown in Fig. 3.2.

The powder metallurgy technique has demonstrated significant effectiveness in the development of porous samples for biomedical applications. Through precise control and fine-tuning of microstructure and porosity, researchers can optimize the degradation kinetics and also achieve the mechanical properties close to that of human bone tissue (Zhang and Cao 2015; Dehghan-Manshadi et al. 2019; Rabeeh et al.

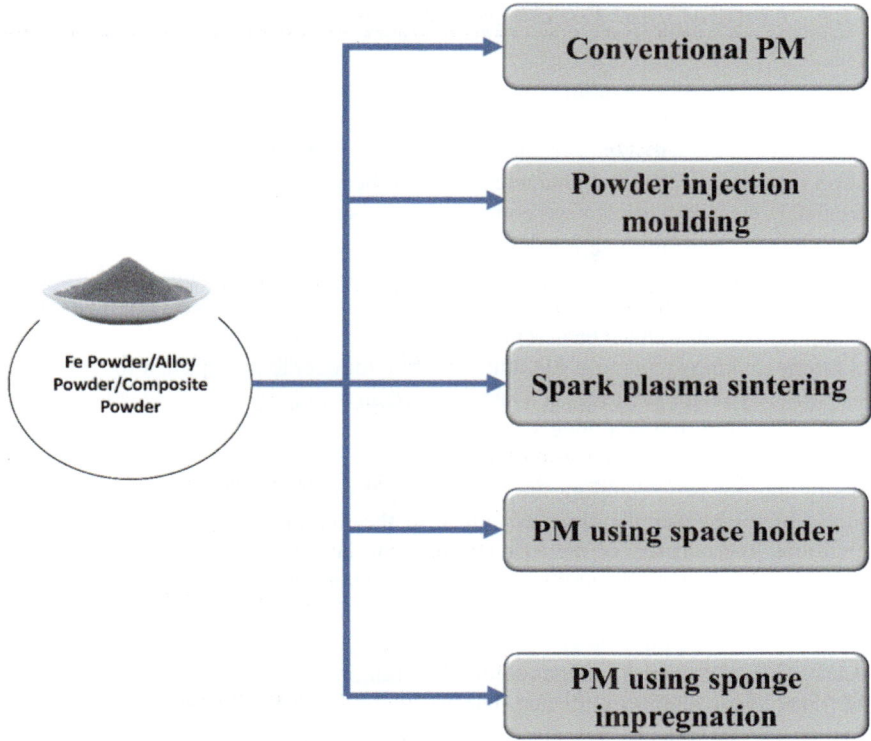

Fig. 3.2 Various powder metallurgical methods

2024a, b). The introduction of a porous morphology serves a dual purpose: it accelerates the rate of degradation and concurrently reduces the elastic modulus of the implant material. This modulation of properties is particularly crucial, as achieving an elastic modulus comparable to that of bone tissue can mitigate the phenomenon of stress shielding. (Ridzwan et al. 2007; Mour et al. 2010; Shayesteh Moghaddam et al. 2016; Prasad et al. 2017). Furthermore, porosity is mostly welcome and considered desirable in implant design due to its multifaceted benefits. A porous structure can facilitate efficient mass transfer of oxygen and nutrients essential for cellular viability and functioning. This can enhance permeability and promotes osseointegration which is essential for the structural and functional correlation between living bone tissue and the implant surface. The porosity can also support vascular invasion considered critical for long-term implant success. Additionally, the increased surface area resulting from porosity can amplify the bioactivity of the implant material. This augmented interfacial area can not only enhance the material's bioactive properties but also improves the mechanical interlocking between the implant and the surrounding tissues, leading to superior fixation and integration (Shimko et al. 2005; Wegener et al. 2020).

3.3.1 Conventional Powder Metallurgy

Conventional powder metallurgy involves several steps: powder production, mixing, compaction, and sintering. This method allows for the direct production of complex shapes and geometries that are often required in implant applications. The degradation rate and mechanical characteristics can be varied significantly by adjusting parameters such as particle size, compaction pressure, and sintering temperature. A schematics of conventional powder metallurgy process is given in Fig. 3.3

Studies have shown that Fe–Mn alloys produced via conventional PM exhibit enhanced degradation rates compared to pure iron. Alloys with varying manganese content (20–35 wt%) have been reported to achieve degradation rates between 1.1 to 1.3 mmpy making them more suitable candidate for degradable application than pure iron, which typically degrades at a rate of less than 0.2 mmpy. Recently cold pressing followed by sintering is a widely used technique for fabricating Fe-based implants (Rabeeh et al. 2022a, 2023). The process allows for precise control over the material's density and porosity, enabling the fine-tuning of the degradation behaviour to suit specific biomedical applications. By adjusting the compaction pressure and sintering conditions, the porosity of the final implant can be optimized, thus directly influencing its mechanical properties and in vitro degradation performance. Figure 3.4 shows the optical micrograph and the pore size distribution of the powder metallurgically prepared pure Fe (Rabeeh et al. 2022a). Hermawan et al. (2008) developed Fe–Mn alloys with manganese content ranging from 20 to 35 wt.% using the PM route. Their findings indicated that these alloys exhibited a significantly higher degradation rate in a physiological environment compared to pure Fe. Specifically, the Fe-20Mn and Fe-25Mn alloys displayed a multiphase microstructure, while the Fe-30Mn and Fe-35Mn alloys consisted of a single-phase microstructure. The multiphase alloys demonstrated a faster degradation rate, ranging from 1.1 to 1.3 mmpy, in contrast to the single-phase alloys, which degraded at a slower rate of 0.4 to 0.7 mmpy. Additionally, the magnetic susceptibility of all alloys was comparable to that of the standard SS316L stainless steel (Hermawan et al. 2010b). Further, Hermawan and Mantovani (2010, 2013) also synthesized Fe–Mn alloys, specifically Fe-25Mn and Fe-35Mn compositions, which exhibited an average degradation rate of 0.5 mmpy—approximately twice that of pure Fe.

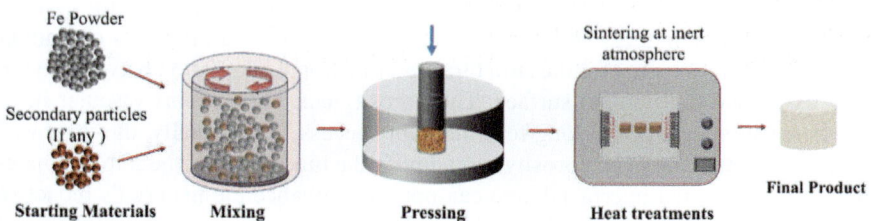

Fig. 3.3 Schematics of conventional powder metallurgy route

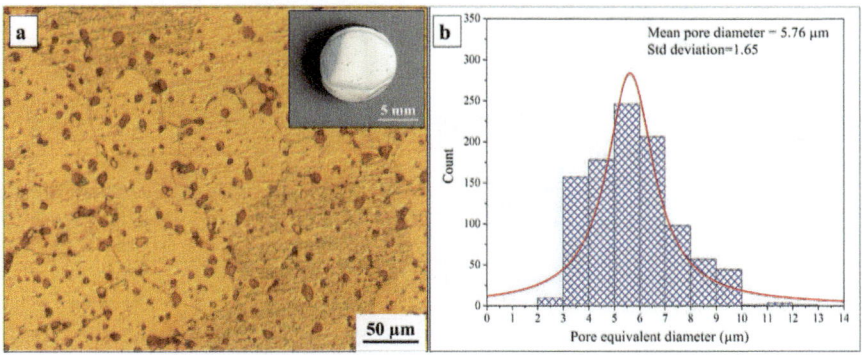

Fig. 3.4 Optical micrograph and the pore size distribution of the powdermetallurgically prepared pure Fe. Reprinted with permission of Elsevier from Rabeeh et al. (2022a)

Wegener et al. (2011) conducted a comprehensive study on a series of low-alloy Fe systems, including Fe-C (0.01 and 0.02 wt.% C), Fe–P (0.6 and 1.6 wt.% P), Fe-B (0.6 wt.% B), and Fe-Ag (1.0 and 5.0 wt.% Ag), synthesized via PM method. The degradation rates of these alloys ranged from 0.123 to 0.187 mmpy, indicating a moderate degradation profile. However, cytotoxicity evaluations revealed that all the alloys, except for the Fe-P systems, exhibited cytotoxicity. Consequently, the study highlighted unalloyed steel and Fe–P alloys as promising candidates for load-bearing implant applications, due to their balanced degradation rates and favourable biocompatibility profiles (Wang et al. 2017).

Powder-metallurgy route was also used for developing metal-matrix composites. Fe / bioceramic composites were developed by many research groups to achieve better biocompatibility and biodegradability (Ulum et al. 2014, 2015; Wang et al. 2017; Rabeeh et al. 2024a, b). Ulum et al. (2014) developed Fe-based composite by incorporating hydroxyapatite (HA), tricalcium phosphate (TCP), and biphasic calcium phosphate (BCP) by mechanical alloying and sintering. Compared with pure-Fe, the composites exhibited a decrease in yield and compressive strength. The incorporation of bioceramic into the Fe matrix also improved its degradation rate. In vitro and in vivo studies revealed that the dispersed bioceramic phase in Fe matrix could improve cell viability and proliferation (Wang et al. 2017; Rabeeh et al. 2024a.).

3.3.2 Powder Injection Moulding

Powder Injection Moulding (PIM) is another advanced PM technique that combines the benefits of injection moulding with powder metallurgy. A schematic of PIM is given in the Fig. 3.5. In this method, metal powders are mixed with a polymer binder to create a feedstock that can be injected into moulds to form complex shapes. After moulding, the binder is removed by heating in controlled environment or treating

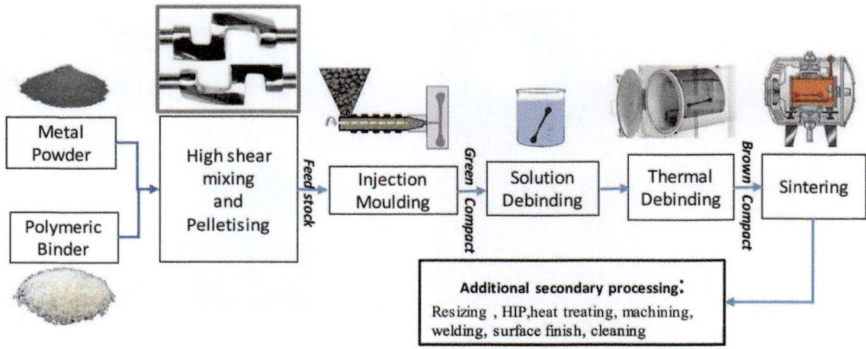

Fig. 3.5 Schematics of powder injection moulding. Reprinted with permission of Elsevier from Dehghan-Manshadi et al. (2020)

with chemical reagents followed by sintering to achieve the desired density and properties.

PIM allows for high production rates and excellent dimensional accuracy, making it suitable for producing intricate implant designs (Demir et al. 2023). However, the challenge lies in ensuring uniform powder dispersion as well as achieving binder removal with no residues and avoiding any compromise in the mechanical properties of the final product.

Tavares et al (2019) and Mariot et al. (2016) fabricated porous pure iron prepared via PIM and reported that the pore structure and porosity significantly influenced the mechanical and surface properties, with higher elongation (up to 50%) and strength values between those of magnesium alloys and 316L stainless steel. The degradation behaviour shifted from pitting corrosion in less dense samples to uniform corrosion in highly densified ones and the in vitro corrosion rate in Hank's solution was higher than of cast iron.

3.3.3 Spark Plasma Sintering

Spark Plasma Sintering (SPS) is an innovative PM technique that uses pulsed electric currents to rapidly sinter powders. This method allows for shorter processing times and lower temperatures compared to traditional sintering methods while achieving high densification. A schematic representation of SPS is given in Fig. 3.6. SPS has been shown to produce Fe-based alloys with fine—grained microstructures that enhance both mechanical properties and degradation rates. For example, Fe–Mn alloys with various elements processed via SPS have demonstrated superior degradation behaviour due to their refined microstructure that facilitates controlled corrosion in physiological environments (Cheng and Zheng 2013; Huang et al. 2014; Montufar et al. 2016).

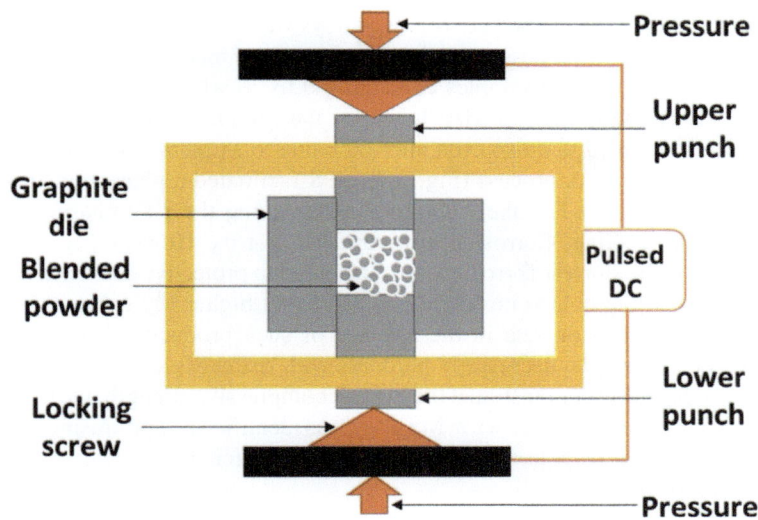

Fig. 3.6 Schematics of spark plasma sintering process Reprinted from Ujah et al. 2023 (CC BY 4.0)

Cheng et al. (2014) developed Fe-Fe2O3 composites using Spark Plasma Sintering (SPS) from Fe-Fe_2O_3 powders containing varying weight percentages (2, 5, 10, 50 wt.%) of Fe_2O_3. The resulting composites exhibited a fine-grained microstructure. The addition of small amounts of Fe_2O_3 (2 and 5 wt.%) significantly enhanced the yield and compressive strength of the material, whereas higher Fe_2O_3 content (50 wt.%) led to a reduction in both yield and ultimate strength. Electrochemical and immersion tests revealed that the Fe-5Fe_2O_3 composite demonstrated a higher degradation rate compared to other compositions. In vitro studies indicated that the composite was non-cytotoxic to ECV304 and L929 cells and exhibited a low haemolysis rate, affirming its biocompatibility. Similarly, Fe-Au and Fe-Ag composites produced by SPS with varying weight percentages of Au and Ag also exhibited improved mechanical properties due to the refined grain structure. Immersion tests showed that these composites degraded approximately 40% faster than pure Fe (Huang et al. 2016).

Montufar et al. (2016) fabricated load-bearing iron–carbon nanotube-tricalcium phosphate (Fe/TCP) composite though SPS. The tensile strength of Fe/TCP composite exhibited a higher value than pure ceramic and comparable to pure iron. Nevertheless, despite the rapid sintering process, partial phase transformation of α-TCP to β-TCP occurred. Carbon nanotubes in the iron powder led to a hypo-eutectoid steel microstructure, and the applied compaction created an anisotropic structure. Though the Fe/TCP surface supported osteoblast adhesion, the local degradation in a confined environment affected cell viability. Further research is needed to refine the sintering conditions, prevent β-TCP formation, and assess long-term degradation behaviour of these composite.

Ueki et al. (2023) developed Fe–Mn–Mg alloys via mechanical alloying and spark plasma sintering (SPS), assessing their degradation and mechanical properties. The findings indicated that the samples containing 0 to 20 wt.% of Mg could achieve a single α(bcc)-phase through MA; however, the samples contains more than 20 wt.% Mg alloys failed to do so even after 60 h due to an increased Mn-to-Fe ratio, which impeded the MA process (Fig. 3.7). SPS facilitated a phase transformation from α-Fe to γ-Fe + ε-Fe, likely due to Mn stabilizing the γ-Fe phase, with ε-Fe forming during cooling. Corrosion tests revealed that the 10 wt.% Mg containing alloy exhibited the slowest corrosion rate, attributed to protective corrosion products on its surface, while polarization tests indicated that higher Mg content correlated with increased corrosion rate in the absence of such products. Vickers hardness measurements showed a decrease in hardness with rising Mg content; nonetheless, the 10 wt.% Mg alloy demonstrated the highest compressive strength due to its lower porosity. Consequently, the 10 wt.% Mg alloy was identified as a promising candidate for Fe-based biodegradable alloys, owing to its superior mechanical strength and moderate corrosion rate.

3.3.4   Powder Metallurgy Using Space Holder

The use of powder metallurgy combined with space holder techniques has emerged as a novel method for fabricating porous materials with controlled porosity, essential for biomedical implants. This approach involves incorporating space holders often made from materials like carbamide, urea, ammonium bicarbonate (NH_4HCO_3) or sodium chloride (NaCl) into a metal powder matrix. During the sintering process, these space holders are removed, leaving behind interconnected pores that enhance the mechanical properties and biocompatibility. A schematic of this technique is given in Fig. 3.8 The studies have shown that using different space holders can yield varying porosity levels and mechanical responses, thus allowing for tailored designs that mimic the natural structure of bone, which is crucial for reducing stress shielding in implants (Čákyová et al. 2024; Čapek and Vojtěch 2014).

Using a space holder which create porosity upon sintering will give the large porosity. Čákyová et al. (2024) reported that biodegradable porous Fe materials, fabricated through powder metallurgy with urea particles serving as space holders, offer a promising and cost-effective biomaterial alternative for the repair of load-bearing bone defects. The mechanical evaluation of these materials through tensile testing revealed that their Young's modulus values were significantly higher than that of natural bone, which is typically around 17 GPa. Electrochemical analysis of corrosion properties demonstrated that samples with a greater number of pores exhibited more negative corrosion potential values, indicating a faster corrosion rate. The sample having highest porosity, displayed the most negative corrosion potential (-622 mV) and the fastest corrosion rate equql to 0.746 mmpy. Additionally, a direct correlation was observed between the quantity of urea used during fabrication and the resulting porosity in the final samples, highlighting a tenable approach to control

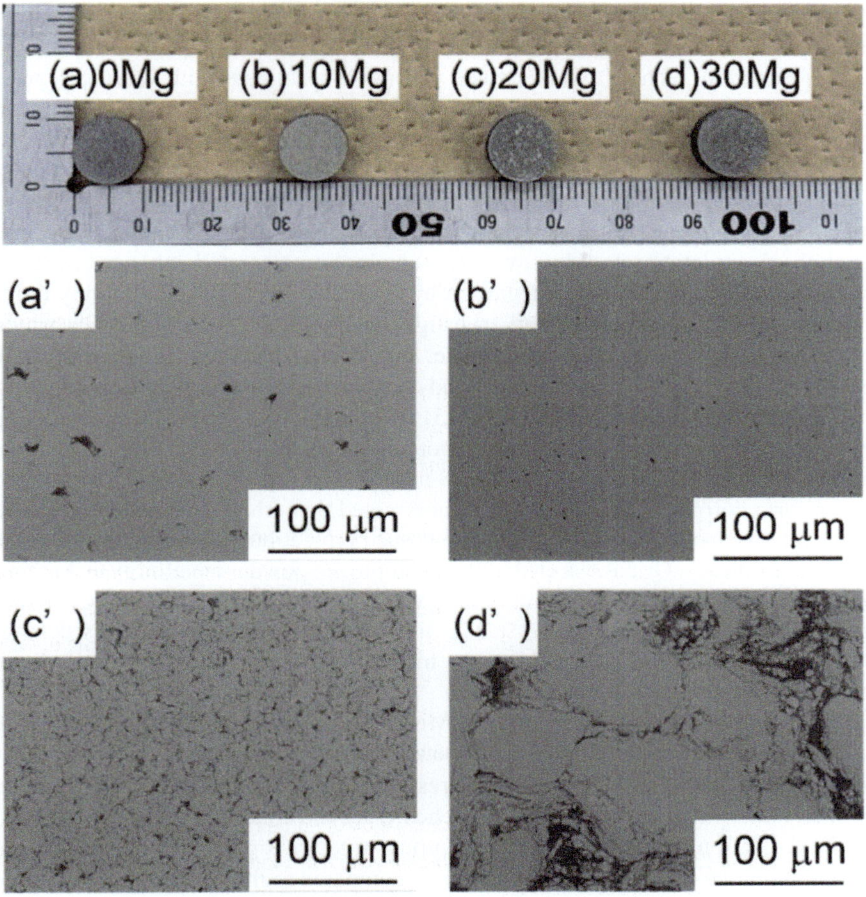

Fig. 3.7 a–c Appearance and (a′, b′, c′) SEM–BSE images of the sintered specimens of (a, a′) 0 Mg, (b, b′) 10 Mg, (c, c′) 20 Mg, and (d, d′) 30 Mg. Reprinted with permission of Elsevier from Ueki et al. (2023)

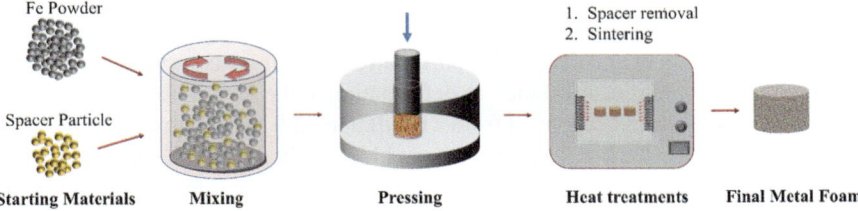

Fig. 3.8 Schematic illustration of fabrication route of metallic scaffold with the space holder method

the corrosion rate by adjusting the amount of urea during the material preparation process.

Čapek and Vojtěch (2014) fabricated porous Fe specimens with varying degrees of porosity utilizing ammonium bicarbonate (NH_4HCO_3) as a space-holding agent. Their findings revealed that the samples predominantly exhibited pore size distributions, ranging from 250 to 500 μm. The authors attributed the formation of smaller pores to insufficient compaction, while the larger pores were generated by the spacer material. The increased surface area provided by the larger pores was found to accelerate the degradation rate. Moreover, the samples demonstrated enhanced biocompatibility and improved osseointegration by facilitating the passage of bodily fluids through the porous structure. This investigation suggests that careful optimization of compaction force, powder particle size, and spacer material selection in iron can enable precise control over porosity and mechanical properties of iron samples. In a similar study, Zhang and Cao (2015) investigated the Fe-35Mn system using NH_4HCO_3 as a space holder, achieving porosity levels of 25–31%. Electrochemical testing revealed a degradation rate of 2–8 mmpy for this porous alloy, characterized by uniform corrosion. However, the authors noted that a high proportion of closed pores relative to open pores may impede tissue permeation, potentially limiting the material's efficacy. Oriňáková et al. (2013a) employed powder metallurgy techniques to generate open-cell porosity in the microstructure of carbonyl iron, Fe-CNT (0.5 wt.% CNT), and Fe–Mg (0.5 wt.% Mg) alloys. Electrochemical analyses demonstrated that the Fe–Mg alloy exhibited a higher degradation rate compared to both pure iron and Fe-CNT compositions.

Heiden et al. (2017) developed Fe–Mn/HA porous composites with two pore sizes, 50 μm and 300 μm. The Fe–Mn powder was blended with NaCl and hydroxyapatite (HA) particles (150 μm), compressed uniaxially, and sintered at 700 °C in an inert atmosphere. After NaCl was leached, a second sintering at 1200 °C resulted in the formation of $Ca_2Mn_7O_{14}$. The porous structure significantly increased the degradation rate of Fe–Mn to 0.79 mm/year compared to the conventional structure (0.24 mm/year). The 300 μm pore size sample, with a degradation rate of 0.82 mm/year, was more favourable for cell adhesion, proliferation, and bone-like apatite biomineralization. These samples also exhibited better mechanical properties than the 50 μm sample, which degraded more rapidly. Similarly, Dehestani et al. (2016) used powder metallurgy to produce Fe-HA composites with varying HA particle sizes (<1 μm, 1–10 μm, and 100–200 μm). Mechanical properties declined with increasing HA content and decreasing particle size. Adding 2.5 wt.% HA halved the yield and tensile strength, attributed to deformation at the HA-Fe interface. With 10 wt.% HA, tensile strength dropped from 213 MPa to 33.9 MPa. The corrosion rate of Fe-HA composites (0.24–1.03 mm/year) was higher than pure Fe (0.11 mm/year), increasing with higher HA content and smaller particle size. Optical images of the sample prepared by PM using space holder technique with different space holding materials are given in Fig. 3.9.

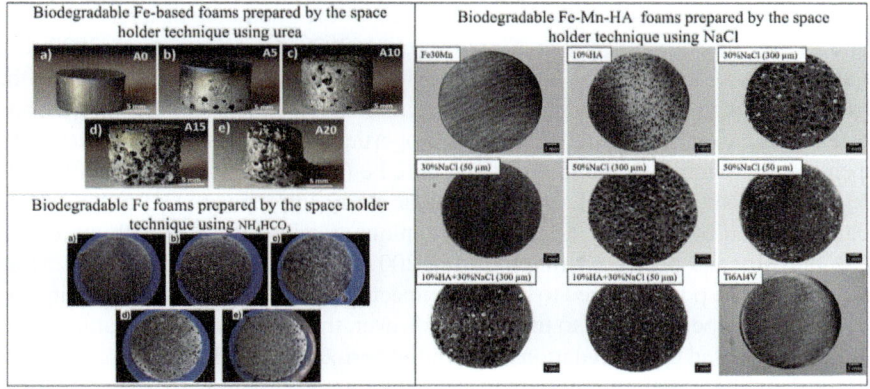

Fig. 3.9 Optical images of the Fe samples prepared by space holder techniques with urea, NH$_4$HCO$_3$ and NaCl as the space holder. Adapted from Čákyová et al. (2024), Čapek J, Vojtěch D (2014), Rabeeh and Hanas (2022b) with permission

3.3.5   Powder Metallurgy Using Sponge Impregnation Technique

Powder metallurgy using sponge impregnation techniques has gained traction for producing open-cell metal foams, particularly due to its ability to create materials that mimic the structure of natural bone. In this process, a polymeric or natural sponge is used as a template, soaked in a slurry of metal powder and a binder. The impregnated sponge is then dried and subjected to a controlled heating process, where the organic material is burned off, and the metal particles sinter together forming a porous metallic structure. The resulting metal foam retains the interconnected, open-cell architecture of the original sponge template, offering high surface area, lightweight, and tailored mechanical properties. Figure 3.10 illustrates the schematic of the sponge impregnation process.

This approach allows for the tailoring of material properties by varying the metal powder composition and processing parameters, making it a versatile method

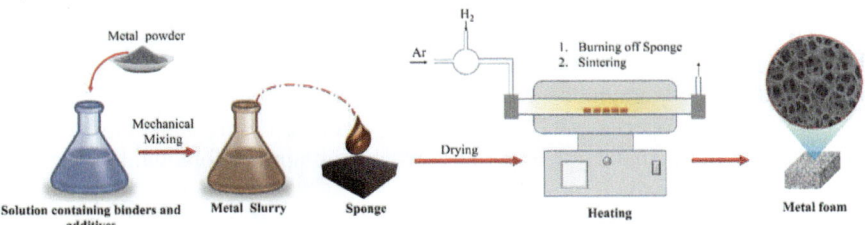

Fig. 3.10   Schematics of powder metallurgy using sponge impregnation technique

for producing lightweight, strong, and biocompatible open-cell structures suitable for various clinical applications (Gorejová et al. 2020; Oriňaková et al. 2020; Liu et al. 2020). Additionally, the interconnected porous (foam) structure can mimic the density of human bone while promoting vascularization which supports nutrient and ion exchange to enhance osteoconductive properties (Rabeeh et al. 2024b). Recently, open cell Fe foams were fabricated from pure Fe (Rabeeh et al. 2024b) and Fe–Mn (53 wt.% of Mn) (Liu et al. 2020) by metal slurry impregnation of polyurethane foam followed by sintering. Using this technique, a microstructure with more than 85% porosity and pore sizes ranging from 200 to 1000 μm were developed. More importantly, the pores seemed to be interconnected, resulting in good bioactivity and mechanical properties close to the bone. However, these highly porous nature of the Fe foam increased the degradation in the initial period and thus need to be controlled. Figure 3.11 shows the morphology of the interconnected porous structure prepared by sponge impregnation and coated with bioactive polymer bioceramic composite to control the degradation rate. The morphology before and after immersion in simulated body fluid shows that the composite coating protects the underlying material and foster biomineralization offering an effective means for preventing initial uncontrolled degradation while enhancing bioactivity.

3.3.6 Processing of Powder Metallurgically Prepared Components

Different thermo-mechanical processing techniques and surface modifications were also adopted while fabricating the components via PM route. These processing can be either during the preparation of samples or after the sintering and are essential for optimizing the performance of degradable iron (Fe) implants in biomedical applications. Techniques such as heat treatment and surface modification can control degradation processes and significantly enhance the mechanical properties as well as biocompatibility of these implants. Heat treatment can be utilized to relieve residual stresses and refine the microstructure, improving strength and ductility, which are critical for load-bearing applications. Surface modifications, including the application of bioactive coatings or surface roughness modifications, can promote osseointegration and enhance corrosion resistance allowing for a more controlled degradation rate that aligns with tissue healing. Additionally, methods like hot isostatic pressing (HIP) can densify the Fe samples, minimizing porosity while maintaining a balance between mechanical integrity and biodegradability. These post-processing strategies are vital for tailoring the properties of PM-prepared degradable Fe implants, ensuring they meet the specific demands of temporary orthopedic applications while promoting safe and effective healing.

Obayi et al. (2015) investigated the effect of rolling on the microstructure, mechanical properties, and degradation behaviour of porous Fe. Their findings indicated that cross-rolled samples exhibited a lower rate of recrystallization compared to

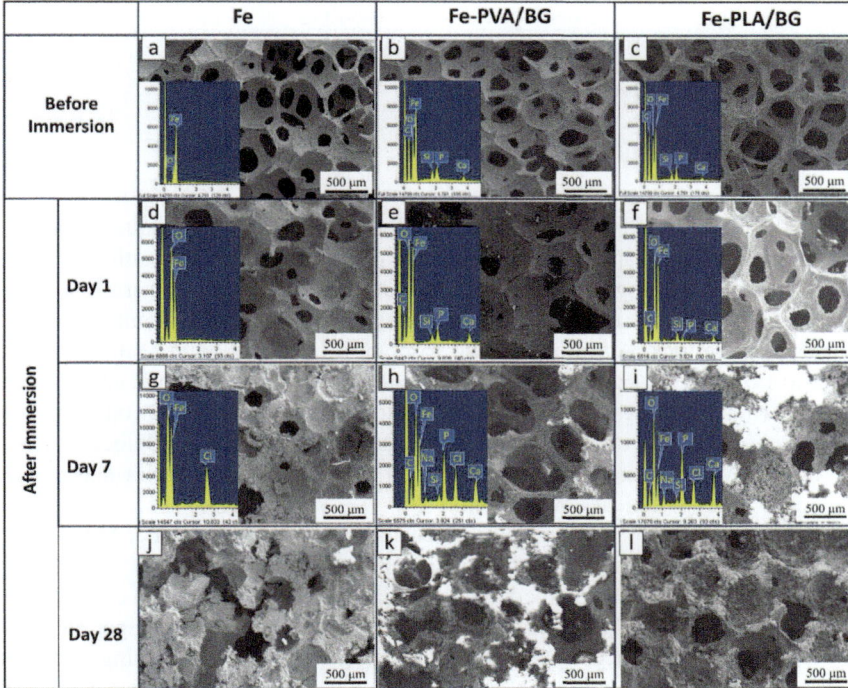

Fig. 3.11 SEM image of the surface morphology of the interconnected porous structure prepared though sponge impregnated method coated with polymer bioceramic composite and their surface morphology after immersion in simulated body. Reprinted with permission of Wiley from Rabeeh et al. (2024b)

straight-rolled samples, primarily due to a reduction in dislocation density, which consequently enhanced the mechanical properties. However, unidirectionally rolled samples showed a higher susceptibility to grain boundary corrosion. In a similar study, Hermawan et al. (2008) employed a cold rolling and sintering approach to fabricate Fe-35Mn alloys from a mixture of Fe and Mn powders. The alloys were subjected to multiple cycles of cold rolling and sintering to improve density. Microstructural analysis revealed the formation of porosity and MnO particles after each cycle. Although sintering was conducted in an inert atmosphere, the air trapped within the micropores likely contributed to the formation of MnO particles (Gierl-Mayer 2020). These cold-rolled samples demonstrated significantly higher degradation rates (0.44–1.26 mmpy) compared to pure annealed Fe, which had a degradation rate of 0.16 mmpy.

Thus, to summarize one can see that there are different approaches that can be explored using the PM metallurgy route. Each of these approaches have its own advantages and disadvantages. Table 3.1 provide a comprehensive summary of the powder metallurgical process used for developing various Fe based degradable implants and the reported in vitro degradation characteristics.

3.4 Casting

Casting as a traditional method is often preferred over other techniques as it helps make intricate shapes and provides better options to alter the composition of alloys. The composition during casting can be optimized by incorporating various alloying elements to accelerate degradation while maintaining sufficient strength for load-bearing applications. Additionally, the formation of a fine grain structure during solidification can be critical for enhancing the corrosion behaviour and mechanical performance of the implant. While casting is advantageous for producing large volumes of implants, one limitation is the formation of internal defects, such as microporosity, which can affect the degradation rate and overall performance of the implant in a physiological environment.

Cheng et al. (2013) investigated the feasibility of as-cast pure Fe, Mn, Mg, Zn and W for use in degradable implants. Their findings indicated that Mg, Zn, and Fe demonstrated favourable biocompatibility, hemocompatibility, and cytocompatibility toward L929 and ECV304 cells. However, defects such as segregation, blowholes, and shrinkage necessitated post-processing techniques, including extrusion, rolling, and forging to modify the microstructure, mechanical properties, and corrosion behaviour. He et al. (2016) reported that cast pure Fe exhibited a degradation rate ranging from 0.105 to 0.29 mmpy. Liu and Zheng (2011) developed binary alloys by incorporating 3 wt.% of elements such as Mn, Co, Al, W, Sn, B, C, and S into Fe. The addition of Mn, Co, Al, W, and B significantly reduced the degradation rate by 50–75%, while the inclusion of C and S had negligible effects in dynamic testing. Although the yield strength of the alloy decreased considerably with the addition of Sn, the other alloying elements slightly enhanced the strength characteristics and increased the gap between yield and ultimate strength of Fe. The extracts from Fe-Co, Mn, Al, W, S, B, C, and S binary alloys exhibited no significant cytotoxicity to ECV304 cells; however, the viability of L929 cells and vascular smooth muscle cells (VSMCs) decreased by 10–15%. All alloys displayed a haemolysis percentage of less than 5%. Additionally, a ternary alloy consisting of 30 wt.% Mn and 6 wt.% silicon (Si) was developed with fine-grained martensite and austenite in the microstructure. This alloy demonstrated a higher degradation rate than pure Fe and Fe–Mn alloys in electrochemical corrosion tests, attributed to the presence of the martensite and austenite phases. The extracts of the Fe-30Mn-6Si alloy initially reduced ECV304 cell viability by 40–50% due to elevated ion release; however, after two days, cell viability improved to 60%. Conversely, VSMC viability declined to nearly 30% (Liu et al. 2011).

Schinhammer et al. (2010, 2013) and Moszner et al. (2011) cast Fe-10Mn-1Pd alloys and applied heat treatment processes, including recrystallization and precipitation, to enhance their microstructural and degradation properties. Heating the alloy to

Table 3.1 Summary of in vitro degradation behaviour of Fe-based BMs developed through various powder metallurgical rout

Materials	Processing method	Degradation medium	Corrosion rate	
			Electrochemical	Static immersion
Fe-W (Cheng and Zheng 2013)	Conventional powder metallurgy	Hank's solution	$1.604–3.025$ $gm^{-2}d^{-1}$	$0.560–0.663$ $gm^{-2}d^{-1}$
Fe-CNT (Cheng and Zheng 2013)	Conventional powder metallurgy	Hank's solution	$2.108–2.419$ $gm^{-2}d^{-1}$	$0.884–1.028$ $gm^{-2}d^{-1}$
Fe–(2–50)Fe$_2$O$_3$ (Cheng et al. 2014)	Conventional powder metallurgy	Hank's solution	$0.107–2.407$ $gm^{-2}d^{-1}$	$0.273–0.668$ $gm^{-2}d^{-1}$
Fe/P	Conventional powder metallurgy	Hank's solution	0.665	–
Fe/P-Mn (Oriňaková et al. 2016)	Conventional powder metallurgy	Hank's solution	2.761 mmpy	–
Fe-2Pd (Čapek et al. 2016b)	Conventional powder metallurgy	SBF	0.43 mmpy	0.787 mmpy
Fe-2Ag (Čapek et al. 2016b)	Conventional powder metallurgy	SBF	0.33 mmpy	0.141 mmpy
Fe-2C (Čapek et al. 2016b)	Conventional powder metallurgy	SBF	0.51 mmpy	0.653 mmpy
Fe-HA (Ulum et al. 2014)	Conventional powder metallurgy	SBF	4.776 $gm^{-2}d^{-1}$	1.008 $gm^{-2}d^{-1}$
Fe-BCP (Ulum et al. 2014)	Conventional powder metallurgy	SBF	4.608 $gm^{-2}d^{-1}$	1.488 $gm^{-2}d^{-1}$
Fe-TCP (Ulum et al. 2014)	Conventional powder metallurgy	SBF	4.344 $gm^{-2}d^{-1}$	2.16 $gm^{-2}d^{-1}$
PLGA incorporated Fe (Yusop et al. 2015)	Conventional powder metallurgy	PBS	–	0.420 mmpy
Fe/Mg$_2$Si (Sikora-Jasinska et al. 2017)	Conventional powder metallurgy	Modified Hank's solution	0.27–0.31 mmpy	0.19–0.28 mmpy
Fe-PE (Gorejová et al. 2020b)	Conventional powder metallurgy	Modified Hank's solution	0.118–0.598 mmpy	0.148–0.697 mmpy

(continued)

Table 3.1 (continued)

Materials	Processing method	Degradation medium	Corrosion rate	
			Electrochemical	Static immersion
Fe-(20–35)Mn (Heiden et al. 2015)	Conventional powder metallurgy	Modified Hank's solution	0.4–1.33 mmpy	-
Porous Fe-30Mn (Dehestani et al. 2017)	Conventional powder metallurgy	SBF	1.36 mmpy	1.18 mmpy
Fe-30Mn (Dehestani et al. 2017)	Conventional powder metallurgy (Heat treated at 700 °C)	SBF	0.29 mmpy	0.24 mmpy
Fe-30Mn (Dehestani et al. 2017)	Conventional powder metallurgy (Annealed at 900 ^{0}C, Quenched)	SBF	0.33 mmpy	0.42 mmpy
PLGA coated Fe (Yusop et al. 2015)	Conventional powder metallurgy (Surface coating)	PBS	–	0.760 mmpy
Pure Fe Rabeeh et al. (2022a)	Conventional powder metallurgy (Au sputtering at the surface)	0.8% NaCl	0.136 mmpy	–
Pure Fe Rabeeh et al. (2022a)	Conventional powder metallurgy	0.8% NaCl	0.402 mmpy	–
Fe-Au composite Rabeeh et al (2023)	Conventional powder metallurgy	0.8% NaCl	0.52–1.35 mmpy	–
Fe-βTCP (Reindl et al. 2014)	Powder injection moulding	0.9%NaCl	–	0.196 mmpy

1250 °C for 12 h in an inert atmosphere, followed by water quenching and isothermal aging below 500 °C, resulted in a 60% increase in degradation rate compared to pure Fe. The formation of Pd-rich precipitates inhibited recrystallization and enhanced mechanical properties through solute drag. Additionally, Obayi et al. (2015) studied cold rolling and annealing effects on as-cast pure Fe, finding that annealed samples exhibited a slight reduction in corrosion rate, attributed to increased average grain size from 16.5 ± 5 μm to 19.6 ± 6 μm. Similarly various post processing techniques were applied for degradable Fe implant made though casting. A Summary of in vitro degradation behaviour of Fe-based BMs developed through casting is given in Table 3.2

3.5 Additive Manufacturing

Additive manufacturing (AM) has emerged as a transformative approach for developing biodegradable Fe implants, enabling the fabrication of complex geometries and tailored porosity that closely resembles natural bone structures. These layer-by-layer fabrication processes facilitate the integration of varying porosity and customized microstructures, which are essential for optimizing the mechanical properties and degradation rates of the implants. Hong et al. (2016) developed porous Fe–Mn scaffolds blended with Ca/Mg using 3D printing, achieving 39.3% and 52.9% porosity with ultimate compressive strengths (UCS) of 228 MPa and 296 MPa, respectively. These scaffolds exhibited a 12-fold higher degradation rate compared to sintered pellets of the same alloys, with the Ca-containing scaffold degrading three times faster. Both showed good biocompatibility with MC3T3 cells. As mentioned in Sect. 3.5, orthopaedic implants need high porosity and permeability to accommodate nutrient perfusion and good cell viability (Nune et al. 2017). However, sometime the large pore size leads to the insufficient mechanical property and low seeding efficiency (Sobral et al. 2011). Yang et al. (2018) developed Fe scaffolds with porosity and UCS (~140 MPa) close to human bone. The optimization of parameters such as layer thickness, scanning speed, and material composition can enhance the bioactivity and mechanical integrity of the resultant implants. Apart from these parameters, the design of the structure also influence the performance. Porous metal scaffolds with Triply Periodic Minimal Surfaces (TPMS), such as diamond, Schwarz, and gyroid structures, are promising for bone scaffold applications. Their design features, including a mean curvature of zero, influence geometric stress concentrations, mechanical properties, and degradation behaviour. Compared to traditional lattices, TPMS offer higher strength-to-weight ratios and larger surface areas, improving bio-integration and affecting degradation rates (Dargusch et al. 2024). These kinds of designs can easily be fabricated though the AM techniques. This methodology represents a promising strategy for the development of innovative, patient-specific iron-based degradable implants. Various types of additive manufacturing rout as detailed in the upcoming sections are explored to develop Fe based degradable implants with desired mechanical properties. (Murr et al. 2010; Zadpoor and Malda 2017; Jiang et al. 2021).

Table 3.2 Summary of in vitro degradation behaviour of Fe-based BMs developed through casting

Materials	Processing method	Degradation medium	Corrosion rate	
			Electrochemical	Static immersion
Pure Fe (Cheng et al. 2013)	Casting	0.9% NaCl	–	0.008 mmpy
Pure Fe (Cheng et al. 2013)	Casting	Hank's solution	–	0.105 mmpy
Pure Fe (Zhu et al. 2009b)	Casting	SBF	–	4.896 $gm^{-2}d^{-1}$
Pure Fe (Moravej et al. 2010b)	Casting (Thermomechanical treated)	Hank's solution	–	0.14 mmpy
Pure Fe (Moravej et al. 2010b)	Casting (Annealed at 550 °C)	Modified Hank's solution	–	0.16 mmpy
Pure Fe (Obayi et al. 2015)	Casting (Rolled)	Modified Hank's solution	0.209–0.243 mmpy	0.115–0.144 mmpy
Fe-20Mn (Chou et al. 2013)	Casting	Osteogenic media	0.9427 mmpy	–
Fe-20Mn (Čapek et al. 2016a)	Casting (Rolled)	Osteogenic media	0.5397 mmpy	–
Fe-30Mn-6Si (Čapek et al. 2016a)	Casting (Rolled)	Hank's solution	–	0.29 mmpy
Fe-Co (Liu and Zheng 2011)	Casting (Rolled)	Hank's solution	2.741–3.025 $gm^{-2}d^{-1}$	0.220–0.250 $gm^{-2}d^{-1}$
Fe-B (Liu and Zheng 2011)	Casting (Rolled)	Hank's solution	2.577–3.741 $gm^{-2}d^{-1}$	0.070–0.142 $gm^{-2}d^{-1}$
Fe-Al (Liu and Zheng 2011)	Casting	Hank's solution	2.385–3.327 $gm^{-2}d^{-1}$	0.116–0.140 $gm^{-2}d^{-1}$
Fe-2Pd (Čapek et al. 2017)	Casting	SBF	–	0.9 $gm^{-2}d^{-1}$
Fe-30Mn (Hufenbach et al. 2018)	Casting (Forged)	SBF	18.91 $gm^{-2}d^{-1}$	0.028 mmpy
Fe-30Mn-1C (Hufenbach et al. 2018)	Casting (Forged)	SBF	–	0.2mmpy
Fe–Mn (Liu and Zheng 2011)	Casting (Forged)	Hank's solution	1.863 $gm^{-2}d^{-1}$	0.028 $gm^{-2}d^{-1}$

3.5.1 Laser Powder Bed Fusion

Laser Powder Bed Fusion (LPBF), also known as Selective Laser Melting (SLM) or Direct Metal Printing (DMP) is a prominent additive manufacturing technique that utilizes a high-energy laser to selectively melt and fuse powdered materials, typically metals, layer by layer to create complex geometries. The process begins with a thin layer of powder spread across a build platform, where the laser selectively targets specific areas to melt the powder, forming a solid layer. This layer is then followed by the application of another powder layer, and the process repeats until the entire part is completed (Fig. 3.12). This additive manufacturing technique allows for the precise construction of complex geometries, which is essential for creating customized implants that fit individual patient anatomies. The printing is done under controlled environments, often using inert gases like argon to prevent oxidation of the metal powders, which ensures high-quality output with desirable mechanical properties.

LPBF excels in producing biodegradable materials, which are particularly promising for orthopedic applications due to their favourable biocompatibility and controlled degradation rates. For instance, LPBF can create intricate porous structures that mimic the mechanical properties of bone, facilitating nutrient transport and promoting tissue regeneration (Liu et al. 2022) Moreover, the rapid melting

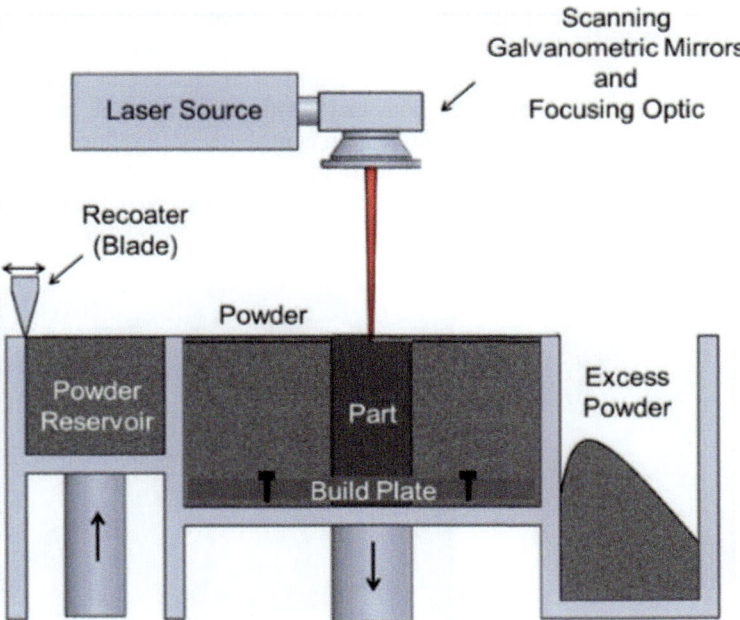

Fig. 3.12 Schematic representation of the laser powder bed fusion (LPBF) process. Reprinted with permission of Elsevier from Gaikwad et al. (2022)

and solidification processes inherent in LPBF enable fine control over microstructural characteristics, which directly influence the mechanical strength and biological response of the implants.

Figure 3.13 shows the porous structure made by the LPBF technique. Nie et al. (2024) fabricated Fe–Mn–Si alloy using LPBF and subjected to annealing treatments. The printed alloy demonstrated superior mechanical properties compared to as cast and annealed counterparts, and cell culture tests confirmed its excellent in vitro biocompatibility, promoting osteoblast proliferation for bone tissue regeneration. Paul et al. (2022) synthesized an Fe-30Mn-1C-0.02S alloy via LPBF and examined the effects of ion release on cell-material interactions. The alloy samples placed in cell culture media for durations of 2 h, 7 days, and 28 days. Notably, cell adhesion remained largely unaffected by the pre-conditioned surfaces during the initial exposure period. Human umbilical vein endothelial cells (HUVECs) were viable for up to 14 days on all three modified surfaces; however, improved cell viability was observed on the degrading sample following 7 and 28 days of pre-conditioning. The authors concluded that the Fe-30Mn-1C-0.02S alloy produced through LPBF exhibits enhanced in vitro biocompatibility, indicating its potential for application in biological environments. Paul et al. (2022) developed an Fe-30Mn-1C-0.02S alloy via laser powder bed fusion (LPBF) and found that pre-conditioned surfaces supported cell survival with better adaptation after 7 and 28 days. The alloy showed improved in vitro biocompatibility suggesting its potential for biomedical use.

Shuai et al. (2019) successfully used SLM technology to fabricate a porous Fe–Mn scaffold, demonstrating the method's precision and versatility in producing metal bone implants with good structural homogeneity and high porosity. The rapid solidification effect of SLM facilitated the dissolution of manganese in the iron matrix resulting in a microstructure with both martensitic and austenitic phases. Additionally, the laser-induced rapid solidification contributed to a refined and uniform microstructure. The mechanical properties of the Fe–Mn scaffold were deemed suitable for load-bearing applications while the degradation rates were found to be faster

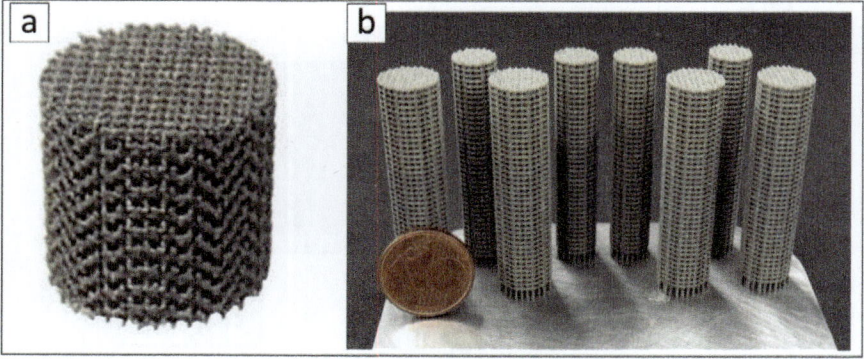

Fig. 3.13 Biodegradable porous Fe structure made by the the the LPBF. Reprinted with permission of Elsevier from Li et al. (2018) and Carluccio et al. (2020)

and more predictable compared to those of pure Fe scaffolds. In vitro cell culture studies confirmed the cytocompatibility of the scaffolds, showing favourable cell proliferation. Similar findings regarding Fe implants developed through SLM were reported by Traverson et al. (2018), Li et al. (2019), and Huang et al. (2021).

Li et al. (2018) developed a topologically ordered, highly porous Fe scaffold using Direct Metal Printing (DMP). The scaffold exhibited a degradation rate approximately 12 times higher than pure Fe in electrochemical tests. After 28 days of in vitro biodegradation in simulated body fluid, its mechanical properties decreased by about 7%, with a weight loss of 3.1%. The enhanced degradation rate was attributed to its porous design. However, direct cell culture with MG-63 cells showed initial cytotoxicity, likely due to high local Fe ion concentrations, which can produce toxic reactive oxygen species. Despite this, the ISO 10993 indirect test confirmed acceptable cytocompatibility in 72-h in vitro assays.

3.5.2 3D Binder Jet Printing

3D binder jet printing has emerged as another promising additive manufacturing technique for the fabrication of degradable metallic implants, offering unique advantages in terms of design flexibility and material processing. This technique can also be used to create porous Fe-based biodegradable materials (Hong et al. 2016; Yang et al. 2018). Like LPBF, 3D binder jet printing also make components layer by layer but by selectively depositing a liquid binding agent onto a powder bed (Fig. 3.14), followed by sintering to achieve the desired design.

Binder jetting offers key advantages over other 3D printing techniques, including high-speed production, versatility with various materials like metals and ceramics, and cost-effectiveness due to reduced waste and energy consumption. It excels in creating intricate designs and complex geometries without the need for support structures, simplifying the production process. These benefits make binder jetting an attractive option for efficient and flexible manufacturing solutions. Recent studies

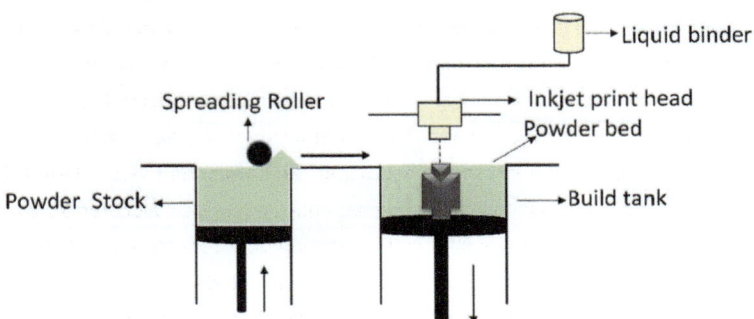

Fig. 3.14 Schematics of binder jet printing. Reprinted from Navaf et al. (2022) under CC BY 4.0

have focused on optimizing binder formulations and post-processing techniques to enhance the mechanical properties of printed iron parts, addressing challenges such as porosity and surface finish. For instance, Rishmawi et al. (2018) highlighted that through careful control of sintering and infiltration processes, it is possible to achieve iron implants with improved strength and biocompatibility, making them suitable for orthopedic applications.

3.5.3 Extrusion-Based 3D Printing

Extrusion-based 3D printing, commonly known as Fused Deposition Modeling (FDM) or Fused Filament Fabrication (FFF), is a widely utilized additive manu-facturing technique that involves the layer-by-layer deposition of material. It can be categorized based on the extrusion mechanism employed, such as filament, plunger or syringe, and screw system. A schematic representation of these three types is provided in Fig. 3.15. In this process, a material composed of metal powders bound in a thermoplastic matrix is heated and extruded through a nozzle, layer by layer, to build the desired part. Once the printing is complete, the resulting "green" part undergoes post-processing steps, including debinding to remove the plastic binder and sintering to fuse the metal particles together into a fully dense component. This method is particularly advantageous due to its affordability and ease of use compared to other metal 3D printing technologies, such as Powder Bed Fusion or Direct Energy Deposition.

Putra et al. (2021) recently created porous iron scaffolds using extrusion-based 3D printing for degradable orthopedic implants. The scaffolds exhibited mechanical

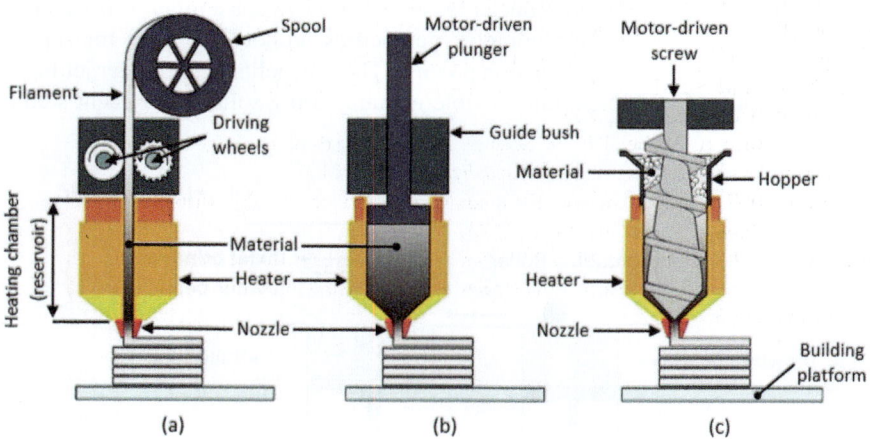

Fig. 3.15 Different types and approaches for extrusion-based additive manufacturing. Reprinted from Gonzalez-Gutierrez eta al. (2018) under CC BY 4.0

Table 3.3 Summary of in vitro degradation behaviour of Fe-based BMs developed through AM

Materials	Processing method	Degradation medium	Corrosion rate	
			Electrochemical	Static immersion
Fe (Čapek et al. 2017)	Additive manufacturing (SPS)	SBF	–	3.20 gm^{-2}d^{-1}
Fe-2Pd (Čapek et al. 2017)	Additive manufacturing (SPS)	SBF	–	0.3 gm^{-2}d^{-1}
Fe-2Pd (Porous)(Čapek et al. 2017)	Additive manufacturing (SPS)	SBF	–	0.8 gm^{-2}d^{-1}
Fe–Mn (Hong et al. 2016)	3D-printed	HBSS	0.04 mmpy	–
Fe–Mn-1Ca (Hermawan et al. 2010b)	3D-printed	HBSS	0.07 mmpy	–
Fe-30Mn (Liu et al. 2011)	3D-printed	HBSS	**mpy**	–

properties, including an elastic modulus of 0.6 GPa, similar to human trabecular bone. After 28 days of static immersion in simulated body fluid (SBF), the scaffold lost 7% of its mass. However, when pre osteoblasts were directly cultured on the scaffold, a significant level of cytotoxicity was observed.

Jiang et al. (2021) utilized FFF to create a Polylactic acid (PLA)/Fe composite scaffold to study its interaction with bone marrow cells. The composite scaffold showed a 15% increase in strut width, an 8% decrease in pore size, and smoother surface texture compared to the PLA scaffold. Additionally, the PLA/Fe composite demonstrated improved hydrophilicity, which contributed to enhanced cell interaction and cytocompatibility.

A Summary of in vitro degradation behaviour of Fe-based BMs developed through AM is given in Table 3.3

3.6 Other Methods

Apart from powder metallurgy, casting and additive manufacturing various other techniques also used to fabricate degradable Fe implant. Some of the techniques are detailed below.

3.6.1   Electroforming

Electroforming is a specialized manufacturing technique that involves the electrodeposition of metal onto a substrate to create complex shapes and structures with high precision. Electroforming offers the unique advantage of fabricating thin-walled cylinders that are free of joint lines (McGeough et al. 2001). This capability cannot be replicated by other manufacturing processes, including casting and powder metallurgy. As a result, this technique could be utilized to create stent mini-tubes and entire stent designs in their final configuration (Moravej et al. 2010a). A solution of $FeCl_2$ and $CaCl_2$ as the electrolyte, known as Fischer–Langbien solution was made by dissolving 400 g of $FeCl_2$ and 80 g of $CaCl_2$ in one liter of deionized water, with additives to reduce stress and prevent corrosion. A polished titanium alloy substrate served to deposit the iron. The solution's pH was adjusted to 1, and the temperature set at 90 °C. Iron was deposited on the substrate for 4.5 h at a current density of 2 A/dm^2, resulting in 100 μm thick iron foils. After deposition, the foils were annealed at 550 °C and 650 °C in an argon atmosphere to relieve internal stresses and enhance ductility.

The fabrication of biodegradable Fe implants, particularly for cardiovascular stents, has seen significant advancements due to this method. It provides the ability to produce iron foils and mini-tubes with we defined microstructures that are required for attaining the desired mechanical properties and degradation rates (Moravej et al. 2010b) The features like fine grains and high yield strength makes it suitable for applications demanding mechanical integrity during implantation. Moreover, the electroforming technique permits the adjustment of factors such as electrolyte composition, current density, and temperature, which can profoundly impact the resulting material properties.

Moravej et al. (2010a) fabricated a thin (~100 μm thick) iron foil on Ti6Al4V alloy surfaces via an electroforming method. After separation from the substrate, the electroformed iron (E-Fe) was annealed in an inert atmosphere. The texture and morphology of the E-Fe were significantly influenced by the process parameters, notably the current density. Annealing resulted in decreased strength and increased elongation due to recrystallization. Initially, E-Fe displayed a degradation rate of 0.85 mm/year, which was greater than that of pure iron, but this rate diminished to 0.51 mm/year after annealing. The higher degradation rate before annealing was attributed to internal stresses and defects present in the as-electroformed state. In a subsequent study, the authors examined how thermomechanical treatment affected E-Fe biodegradation and cytocompatibility. Both static and dynamic immersion tests confirmed that E-Fe had not only enhanced degradation without thermomechanical treatment but also demonstrated good compatibility with rat smooth muscle cells fostering enhanced cell proliferation (Moravej et al. 2010b).

Further studies by Moravej et al. (2011) evaluated how current density influences the microstructure and biodegradability of iron deposited on titanium using electrodeposition. Four different current densities (1, 2, 5, and 10 A/dm^2) were applied, and it was observed that the grain size, shape, and texture of the electroformed iron were heavily influenced by the current density. In corrosion tests, the iron deposited at 2 A/dm^2 corroded the least, followed by those deposited at 10, 1, and 5 A/dm^2. However, after 14 days of immersion in HBSS all samples showed similar degradation rates, which was attributed to the formation of a passivation layer. The authors suggested that electroformed iron, due to the presence of micro pits, could be advantageous for use in biodegradable implants as these pits promote faster degradation.

3.6.2 Magnetron Sputtering

Magnetron sputtering is an advanced deposition technique that has gained attention for its application in creating biodegradable iron implants. This method utilizes a high-energy plasma to eject atoms from a target material, which then deposit onto a substrate, forming thin films with controlled thickness and composition. In the context of Fe-based biodegradable implants, magnetron sputtering enables the fabrication of structured Fe–Mn foils, which exhibit enhanced mechanical properties and biocompatibility due to the addition of manganese (Jurgeleit et al. 2015, 2016).

Jurgeleit et al. (2015, 2016) used magnetron sputtering, and UV lithography for developing Au sputtered Fe multi-layered foils. The process was tuned to provide a microstructure with Au incorporated between the Fe layers. Three different samples with Au content 0.3, 1 and 2.5 at% was developed in this work. The introduction of Au enhanced the degradation rate of the foils significantly. It is reported that the samples with 1at% Au exhibit the best compromise between low Au content, mechanical properties and degradation rate. The authors suggested that the precision of this method can help to fabricate devices with a gradient in the microstructure composition. Using this approach, the degradation rate during the initial implantation period can be slowed down to maintain mechanical integrity and promote better implant-tissue interaction. Such a system can be achieved by fine-tuning the process to incorporate a lesser amount of gold on the surface compared to the core of the implant.

Another study by Jurgeleit et al. (2017) demonstrates that freestanding Fe–FeMn32 multilayer films can be successfully deposited using magnetron sputtering, followed by post-deposition annealing to achieve a fine-grained, recrystallized microstructure. The Mn content significantly influences both the phase composition and material behaviour. Films with Mn content up to 10 wt % exhibit an α'-phase, while higher Mn levels (15–17 wt %) show γ- and ϵ-phases. As Mn concentration increases, ferromagnetic behaviour decreases, and strength improves while ductility is reduced. FeMn15 and FeMn17 were found to offer an optimal balance between high strength, sufficient ductility, and non-ferromagnetic behaviour, making them suitable for MRI-compatible implants. The fine microstructure produced via magnetron sputtering allows for high strength and eliminates the need for additional processing steps that could alter material properties. Despite a low degradation rate, the relative surface area of an implant can be increased to compensate, making this fabrication technique advantageous for biomedical applications.

Table 3.4 Advantages and disadvantages of the various method for manufacturing Fe-based biodegradable devices. Reprinted with permission of Springer Nature from Rabeeh and Hanas (2022b)

Method	Advantages	Disadvantages
Powder Metallurgy	• Allows the direct production of relatively complex shapes • Materials with tuned properties can be obtained • The degradation rate and mechanical characteristics can be varied across a large range by making minor modifications to production parameters • A suitable method for developing alloys, composites, and porous materials • Ease of tailoring biodegradability by optimising porosity	• Difficulties in powder preparation • Chances of inhomogeneity during the mixing/milling process leads to poor mechanical properties
Casting	• Affordability of alloys • Composition customization • Easy to make complicated geometry	• There is a high probability of casting defects such as segregation, blowholes, and shrinkage • Post-processing is required after casting • Difficult to produce Fe-bioceramic composite • High-stress shielding
Additive manufacturing	• Best method to produce porous scaffolds • Ease of tailoring biodegradability by optimising porosity • Shape and geometry of the pores can be controlled (these decide the osseocunduction and osseointegration • Allows implant materials to have mechanical characteristics similar to human bone. (Reduce stress shielding) • Accuracy and adaptability	• Difficulties in powder preparations
Electroforming	• Simple method • Does not require complex equipment • Less amount of energy consumption	• Only thin sections/sheets can be made

To summarise the chapter one can note that there are various manufacturing routes possible for developing degradable metallic implants using Fe. Each techniques have their own merits and demerits. While some routes follow conventional routes, the recently added techniques explores the possibility of advancements in technology for materials fabrication. The advantages and disadvantages of the various method for manufacturing Fe-based biodegradable devices reported so far are listed in Table 3.4.

References

Čákyová V, Gorejová R, Macko R, Petruš O, Sopčák T, Kupková M et al (2024) Biodegradable iron-based foams prepared by the space holder technique using urea. J Appl Electrochem 54:625–634. https://doi.org/10.1007/s10800-023-01993-x

Čapek J, Vojtěch D (2014) Microstructural and mechanical characteristics of porous iron prepared by powder metallurgy. Mater Sci Eng C 43:494–501. https://doi.org/10.1016/j.msec.2014.06.046

Carluccio D, Xu C, Venezuela J, Cao Y, Kent D, Bermingham M, Demir AG, Previtali B, Ye Q, Dargusch M (2020) Additively manufactured iron-manganese for biodegradable porous load-bearing bone scaffold applications. Acta Biomater 103:346–360. https://doi.org/10.1016/j.actbio.2019.12.018

Cheng J, Huang T, Zheng YF (2014a) J Biomed Mater Res A 102:2277–2287. https://doi.org/10.1002/jbm.a.34882

Cheng J, Zheng YF (2013) In vitro study on newly designed biodegradable Fe-X composites (X = W, CNT) prepared by spark plasma sintering. J Biomed Mater Res B Appl Biomater 101:485–497. https://doi.org/10.1002/jbm.b.32783

Dargusch MS, Soro N, Demir AG, Venezuela J, Sun Q, Wang Y et al (2024) Optimising degradation and mechanical performance of additively manufactured biodegradable Fe–Mn scaffolds using design strategies based on triply periodic minimal surfaces. Smart Mater Med 5:127–139. https://doi.org/10.1016/j.smaim.2023.10.003

Dehestani M, Adolfsson E, Stanciu LA (2016) Mechanical properties and corrosion behavior of powder metallurgy iron-hydroxyapatite composites for biodegradable implant applications. Mater des 109:556–569. https://doi.org/10.1016/j.matdes.2016.07.092

Dehghan-Manshadi A, StJohn DH, Dargusch MS (2019) Tensile properties and fracture behaviour of biodegradable iron-manganese scaffolds produced by powder sintering. Materials 12. https://doi.org/10.3390/ma12101572

Dehghan-Manshadi A, Yu P, Dargusch M, StJohn D, Qian M (2020) Metal injection moulding of surgical tools, biomaterials and medical devices: a review. Powder Technol 364:189–204. https://doi.org/10.1016/j.powtec.2020.01.073

Demir G, Akyurek D, Hassoun A, Mutlu I (2023) Production of biodegradable metal foams by powder metallurgy method. Phys Mesomech 26:196–208. https://doi.org/10.1134/S10299599 2302008X

Gaikwad A, Williams RJ, de Winton H, Bevans BD, Smoqi Z, Rao P, Hooper PA (2022) Multi-phenomena melt pool sensor data fusion for enhanced process monitoring of laser powder bed fusion additive manufacturing. Mater des 221:110919. https://doi.org/10.1016/j.matdes.2022.110919

Gierl-Mayer C (2020) Reactions between ferrous powder compacts and atmospheres during sintering—an overview 63:237–253. https://doi.org/10.1080/00325899.2020.1810427

Gonzalez-Gutierrez J, Cano S, Schuschnigg S, Kukla C, Sapkota J, Holzer C (2018) Additive manufacturing of metallic and ceramic components by the material extrusion of highly-filled polymers: a review and future perspectives. Materials 11:840. https://doi.org/10.3390/ma1105 0840

Gorejová R, Oriňaková R, Orságová Králová Z et al (2020) In vitro corrosion behavior of biodegradable iron foams with polymeric coating. Materials (Basel) 13:1–17. https://doi.org/10.3390/ma1 3010184

He J, He F, Li D, et al (2016) Advances in Fe-based biodegradable metallic materials. RSC Adv, 112819–112838.https://doi.org/10.1039/c6ra20594a

Heiden M, Nauman E, Stanciu L (2017) Bioresorbable Fe–Mn and Fe–Mn–HA materials for orthopedic implantation: enhancing degradation through porosity control. Adv Healthc Mater 6:1700120. https://doi.org/10.1002/ADHM.201700120

Hermawan H, Alamdari H, Mantovani D, Dubé D (2008) Iron–manganese: new class of metallic degradable biomaterials prepared by powder metallurgy. Powder Metall 51:38–45. https://doi.org/10.1179/174329008X284868

Hermawan H, Dubé D, Mantovani D (2010a) Degradable metallic biomaterials: design and development of Fe-Mn alloys for stents. J Biomed Mater Res A 93:1–11. https://doi.org/10.1002/jbm.a.32224

Hermawan H, Mantovani D (2013) Process of prototyping coronary stents from biodegradable Fe-Mn alloys. Acta Biomater 9:8585–8592. https://doi.org/10.1016/j.actbio.2013.04.027

Hermawan H, Purnama A, Dube D et al (2010b) Fe-Mn alloys for metallic biodegradable stents: degradation and cell viability studies. Acta Biomater 6:1852–1860. https://doi.org/10.1016/j.actbio.2009.11.025

Hong D, Chou DT, Velikokhatnyi OI et al (2016) Binder-jetting 3D printing and alloy development of new biodegradable Fe-Mn-Ca/Mg alloys. Acta Biomater 45:375–386. https://doi.org/10.1016/j.actbio.2016.08.032

Huang CC, Lam TN, Amalia L et al (2021) Tailoring grain sizes of the biodegradable iron-based alloys by pre-additive manufacturing microalloying. Sci Rep 11. https://doi.org/10.1038/S41598-021-89022-9

Huang T, Cheng J, Zheng YF (2014) In vitro degradation and biocompatibility of Fe-Pd and Fe-Pt composites fabricated by spark plasma sintering. Mater Sci Eng, C 35:43–53. https://doi.org/10.1016/j.msec.2013.10.023

Huang T, Cheng Y, Zheng Y (2016) In vitro studies on silver implanted pure iron by metal vapor vacuum arc technique. Colloids Surf B Biointerfaces 142:20–29. https://doi.org/10.1016/j.colsurfb.2016.01.065

Jiang D, Ning F, Wang Y (2021) Additive manufacturing of biodegradable iron-based particle reinforced polylactic acid composite scaffolds for tissue engineering. J Mater Process Technol 289:116952. https://doi.org/10.1016/J.JMATPROTEC.2020.116952

Jurgeleit T, Quandt E, Zamponi C (2015) Magnetron sputtering a new fabrication method of iron based biodegradable implant materials. Adv Mater Sci Eng 2015:1–9. https://doi.org/10.1155/2015/294686

Jurgeleit T, Quandt E, Zamponi C (2016) Mechanical properties and in vitro degradation of sputtered biodegradable Fe-Au foils. Materials 9:928. https://doi.org/10.3390/ma9110928

Jurgeleit T, Quandt E, Zamponi C (2017) Magnetron sputtering as a fabrication method for a biodegradable Fe32Mn alloy. Materials 10:1196. https://doi.org/10.3390/ma10101196

Li Y, Jahr H, Lietaert K et al (2018) Additively manufactured biodegradable porous iron. Acta Biomater 77:380–393. https://doi.org/10.1016/j.actbio.2018.07.011

Li Y, Jahr H, Pavanram P et al (2019) Additively manufactured functionally graded biodegradable porous iron. Acta Biomater 96:646–661. https://doi.org/10.1016/j.actbio.2019.07.013

Liu B, Zheng YF (2011) Effects of alloying elements (Mn Co, Al, W, Sn, B, C and S) on biodegradability and in vitro biocompatibility of pure iron. Acta Biomater 7:1407–1420. https://doi.org/10.1016/J.ACTBIO.2010.11.001

Liu B, Zheng YF, Ruan L (2011) In vitro investigation of Fe30Mn6Si shape memory alloy as potential biodegradable metallic material. Mater Lett 65:540–543. https://doi.org/10.1016/j.matlet.2010.10.068

Liu C, Ling C, Chen C, Wang D, Yang Y, Xie D, Shuai C (2022) Laser additive manufacturing of magnesium alloys and its biomedical applications. Mater Sci Addit Manuf 1:24. https://doi.org/10.18063/msam.v1i4.24

Liu P, Zhang D, Dai Y et al (2020) Microstructure, mechanical properties, degradation behavior, and biocompatibility of porous Fe-Mn alloys fabricated by sponge impregnation and sintering techniques. Acta Biomater 114:485–496. https://doi.org/10.1016/j.actbio.2020.07.048

Mariot P, Leeflang MA, Schaeffer L, Zhou J (2016) An investigation on the properties of injection-molded pure iron potentially for biodegradable stent application. Powder Technol 294:226–235. https://doi.org/10.1016/j.powtec.2016.02.042

McGeough JA, Leu MC, Rajurkar KP, De Silva AKM, Liu Q (2001) Electroforming process and application to micro/macro manufacturing. CIRP Ann 50:499–514. https://doi.org/10.1016/S0007-8506(07)62990-4

Montufar EB, Horynová M, Casas-Luna M et al (2016) Spark plasma sintering of load-bearing iron-carbon nanotube-tricalcium phosphate cermets for orthopaedic applications. JOM 68:1134–1142. https://doi.org/10.1007/S11837-015-1806-9/FIGURES/8

Moravej M, Amira S, Prima F, et al (2011) Effect of electrodeposition current density on the microstructure and the degradation of electroformed iron for degradable stents. In: Materials science and engineering B: solid-state materials for advanced technology. Elsevier B.V., pp 1812–1822

Moravej M, Prima F, Fiset M, Mantovani D (2010a) Electroformed iron as new biomaterial for degradable stents: Development process and structure-properties relationship. Acta Biomater 6:1726–1735. https://doi.org/10.1016/j.actbio.2010.01.010

Moravej M, Purnama A, Fiset M, et al (2010b) Electroformed pure iron as a new biomaterial for degradable stents: In vitro degradation and preliminary cell viability studies. Acta Biomater 6:1843–1851. https://doi.org/10.1016/j.actbio.2010.01.008

Moszner F, Sologubenko AS, Schinhammer M et al (2011) Precipitation hardening of biodegradable Fe-Mn-Pd alloys. Acta Mater 59:981–991. https://doi.org/10.1016/j.actamat.2010.10.025

Mour M, Das D, Winkler T, et al (2010) Advances in porous biomaterials for dental and orthopaedic applications. Materials 3:2947–2974. https://doi.org/10.3390/MA3052947

Murr LE, Gaytan SM, Medina F et al (2010) Next-generation biomedical implants using additive manufacturing of complex, cellular and functional mesh arrays. Philos Trans Royal Soc A Mathem Phys Eng Sci 368:1999–2032. https://doi.org/10.1098/rsta.2010.0010

Navaf M, Sunooj KV, Aaliya B, Akhila PP, Sudheesh C, Mir SA, George J (2022) 4D printing: a new approach for food printing; effect of various stimuli on 4D printed food properties. a comprehensive review. Appl Food Res 2:100150. https://doi.org/10.1016/j.afres.2022.100150

Nie Y, Yuan B, Liang J, Deng T, Li X, Chen P, Zhang K, Li X, Li K, Peng H, Gong S (2024) Mechanical and functional properties of Fe–Mn–Si biodegradable alloys fabricated by laser powder bed fusion: effect of heat treatment. Mater Sci Eng A 908:146725. https://doi.org/10.1016/j.msea.2024.146725

Nune KC, Kumar A, Misra RDK et al (2017) Functional response of osteoblasts in functionally gradient titanium alloy mesh arrays processed by 3D additive manufacturing. Colloids Surf B Biointerfaces 150:78–88. https://doi.org/10.1016/j.colsurfb.2016.09.050

Obayi CS, Tolouei R, Paternoster C et al (2015) Influence of cross-rolling on the micro-texture and biodegradation of pure iron as biodegradable material for medical implants. Acta Biomater 17:68–77. https://doi.org/10.1016/j.actbio.2015.01.024

Oriňaková R, Gorejová R, Králová ZO, Oriňak A (2020) Surface modifications of biodegradable metallic foams for medical applications. Coatings 10. https://doi.org/10.3390/coatings10090819

Oriňaková R, Oriňak A, Giretová M et al (2016) A study of cytocompatibility and degradation of iron-based biodegradable materials. J Biomater Appl 30:1060–1070. https://doi.org/10.1177/0885328215615459

Paul B, Lode A, Placht AM, et al (2022) Cell-material interactions in direct contact culture of endothelial cells on biodegradable iron-based stents fabricated by laser powder bed fusion and impact of ion release. ACS Appl Mater Interfaces 14:439–451. https://doi.org/10.1021/acsami.1c21901

Prasad K, Bazaka O, Chua M, et al (2017) Metallic biomaterials: current challenges and opportunities. Materials 10.https://doi.org/10.3390/MA10080884

Rabeeh VPM, Hanas T (2022a) Enhancing biointerfacial properties of porous pure iron by gold sputtering for degradable implant applications. Mater Today Commun 31:103492. https://doi.org/10.1016/J.MTCOMM.2022.103492

Rabeeh VPM, Hanas T (2022b) Progress in manufacturing and processing of degradable Fe-based implants: a review. Progress in Biomaterials 11:2 11:163–191. https://doi.org/10.1007/S40204-022-00189-4

Rabeeh VM, Rahim SA, Kinattingara Parambath S, Rajanikant GK, Hanas T (2023) Iron–gold composites for biodegradable implants: in vitro investigation on biodegradation and biomineralization. ACS Biomater Sci Eng 9:4255–4268. https://doi.org/10.1021/acsbiomaterials.3c00513

Rabeeh VPM, Surendramohan KS, Jyothis S et al (2024a) Fostering biomineralization and biodegradation: nano-hydroxyapatite reinforced iron composites for biodegradable implant application. Discov Mater 4:39. https://doi.org/10.1007/s43939-024-00113-6

Rabeeh VM, Surendramohan KS, Tharayil H (2024b) Bioactive Fe foam for degradable bone graft cages. Adv Eng Mater 26:2301416. https://doi.org/10.1002/adem.202301416

Ridzwan MIZ, Shuib S, Hassan AY et al (2007) Problem of stress shielding and improvement to the hip implant designs: A review. J Med Sci 7:460–467. https://doi.org/10.3923/JMS.2007.460.467

Rishmawi I, Salarian M, Vlasea M (2018) Tailoring green and sintered density of pure iron parts using binder jetting additive manufacturing. Addit Manuf 24:508–520. https://doi.org/10.1016/j.addma.2018.10.015

Schinhammer M, Hänzi AC, Löffler JF, Uggowitzer PJ (2010) Design strategy for biodegradable Fe-based alloys for medical applications. Acta Biomater 6:1705–1713. https://doi.org/10.1016/j.actbio.2009.07.039

Schinhammer M, Steiger P, Moszner F et al (2013) Degradation performance of biodegradable FeMnC(Pd) alloys. Mater Sci Eng, C 33:1882–1893. https://doi.org/10.1016/j.msec.2012.10.013

Shayesteh Moghaddam N, Taheri Andani M, Amerinatanzi A, et al (2016) Metals for bone implants: safety, design, and efficacy. Biomanuf Rev 1:1 1:1–16. https://doi.org/10.1007/S40898-016-0001-2

Shimko DA, Shimko VF, Sander EA, et al (2005) Effect of porosity on the fluid flow characteristics and mechanical properties of tantalum scaffolds. J Biomed Mater Res B Appl Biomater 73:315–324. https://doi.org/10.1002/JBM.B.30229

Shuai C, Yang W, Yang Y et al (2019) Selective laser melted Fe-Mn bone scaffold: microstructure, corrosion behavior and cell response. Mater Res Express 7. https://doi.org/10.1088/2053-1591/AB62F5

Sobral JM, Caridade SG, Sousa RA et al (2011) Three-dimensional plotted scaffolds with controlled pore size gradients: Effect of scaffold geometry on mechanical performance and cell seeding efficiency. Acta Biomater 7:1009–1018. https://doi.org/10.1016/j.actbio.2010.11.003

Tavares AC, Mariot P, Costa LL, Schaeffer L (2019) Metal injection molding for production of biodegradable implants: an analysis of the potential of pure iron for application in stents. Am J Mater Sci 9:36–43. https://doi.org/10.5923/j.materials.20190902.02

Traverson M, Heiden M, Stanciu LA et al (2018) In Vivo Evaluation of Biodegradability and Biocompatibility of Fe30Mn Alloy. Veterinary Comparative Orthopaedics Traumatol 31:10–16. https://doi.org/10.3415/VCOT-17-06-0080

Ueki K, Hirano R, Nakai M (2023) Development of biodegradable Fe–Mn–Mg alloys by mechanical alloying and spark plasma sintering. Mater Today Commun 34:105465. https://doi.org/10.1016/j.mtcomm.2023.105465

Ujah CO, Kallon DVV, Aigbodion VS (2023) High entropy alloys prepared by spark plasma sintering: Mechanical and thermal properties. Mater Today Sustain 100639. https://doi.org/10.1016/j.mtsust.2023.100639

Ulum MF, Arafat A, Noviana D et al (2014) In vitro and in vivo degradation evaluation of novel iron-bioceramic composites for bone implant applications. Mater Sci Eng C 36:336–344. https://doi.org/10.1016/j.msec.2013.12.022

Ulum MF, Nasution AK, Yusop AH et al (2015) Evidences of in vivo bioactivity of Fe-bioceramic composites for temporary bone implants. J Biomed Mater Res B Appl Biomater 103:1354–1365. https://doi.org/10.1002/jbm.b.33315

Wang S, Xu Y, Zhou J et al (2017) In vitro degradation and surface bioactivity of iron-matrix composites containing silicate-based bioceramic. Bioact Mater 2:10–18. https://doi.org/10.1016/j.bioactmat.2016.12.001

Wegener B, Sichler A, Milz S et al (2020) Development of a novel biodegradable porous iron-based implant for bone replacement. Sci Rep 10:1–10. https://doi.org/10.1038/s41598-020-66289-y

Wegener B, Sievers B, Utzschneider S, et al (2011) Microstructure, cytotoxicity and corrosion of powder-metallurgical iron alloys for biodegradable bone replacement materials. In: Materials science and engineering B: solid-state materials for advanced technology. Elsevier B.V., pp 1789–1796

Yang C, Huan Z, Wang X et al (2018) 3D printed Fe scaffolds with HA nanocoating for bone regeneration. ACS Biomater Sci Eng 4:608–616. https://doi.org/10.1021/acsbiomaterials.7b00885

Zadpoor AA, Malda J (2017) Additive manufacturing of biomaterials, tissues, and organs. Ann Biomed Eng 45:1–11. https://doi.org/10.1007/s10439-016-1719-y

Zhang Q, Cao P (2015) Degradable porous Fe-35wt.%Mn produced via powder sintering from NH4HCO3 porogen. Mater Chem Phys 163:394–401. https://doi.org/10.1016/j.matchemphys.2015.07.056

Zheng YF, Gu XN, Witte F (2014) Biodegradable metals. Mater Sci Eng R Rep 77:1–34

Chapter 4
Biodegradable Fe: Processing Techniques

4.1 Introduction

Beyond the traditional and advanced manufacturing techniques outlined in the previous chapter, a variety of metallurgical and surface modification strategies are being employed to adjust the degradation behavior of Fe-based alloys. As illustrated in Fig. 4.1, these strategies can be categorized into alloying, microstructural alterations, and surface modifications. Numerous studies have investigated the potential of enhancing the degradation rate of Fe-based systems through alloying with more noble metals like Mn, Au, and Ag, taking advantage of their differing electrochemical potentials. The focus of microstructure modification has been primarily on creating multiphase structures, which are anticipated to degrade at a faster rate compared to single-phase alloys. Surface modification techniques encompass approaches such as applying coatings for initial stability during implantation, depositing noble metals to establish micro-galvanic cells, and employing chemical processing for surface conversions.

4.2 Alloying

Alloying in Fe-based materials for degradable implant applications plays a crucial role in enhancing their performance, particularly in terms of degradation rates and mechanical properties. Research so far has primarily centered on using Mn as an alloying material (Gorejová et al. 2019), while additional elements such as Pd, C, B, Ag, Si, W, N, Co, Al, Sn, S, Pt, CNTs, Mg, Ga, and Zn have also been studied Rabeeh and Hanas (2022a, b). Biosafety is the primary concers when developing a metallic implant. Thus choosing appropriate alloying element is highly important. Majorly the Fe based alloy system can be classified into Fe–Mn-X system, Fe–X system, Fe–N system and other system.

© The Author(s), under exclusive license to Springer Nature Switzerland AG 2025
VP. Md. Rabeeh and T. Hanas, *Biodegradable Iron Implants: Development, Processing, and Applications*, SpringerBriefs in Materials,
https://doi.org/10.1007/978-3-031-82099-1_4

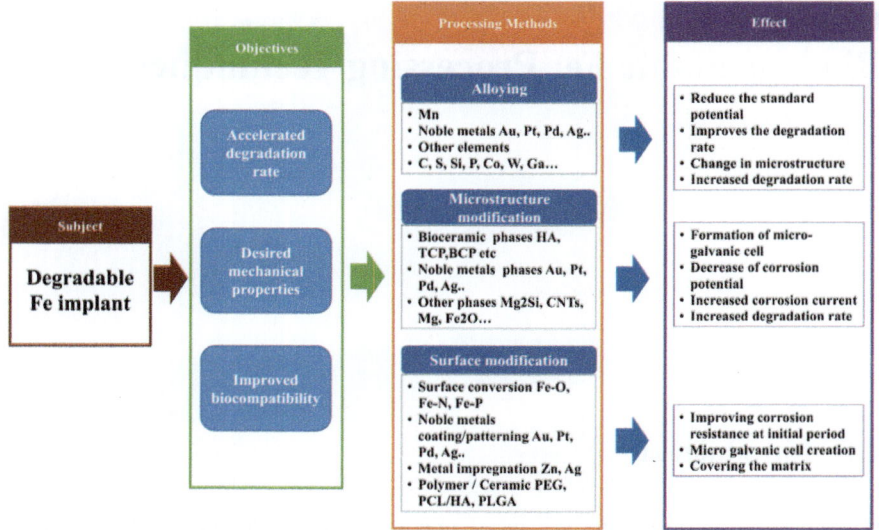

Fig. 4.1 Various processing techniques and method to improve the degradation rate of Fe

4.2.1 Fe–Mn Alloy System

The incorporation of Mn into biodegradable Fe alloys significantly enhances their degradation properties, making them suitable for temporary implant applications. Besides, Mn is a trace element essential for the growth, development and regeneration of healthy bone tissues and several enzyme systems (Beattie and Avenell 1992). Thus, Fe–Mn alloy received much interest, and Mn is now considered a preferred alloying element in the Fe matrix for BMs. Mn lowers the standard electrode potential of the Fe matrix, which results in an increased corrosion rate compared to pure Fe. Research indicates that an optimal Mn content of around 30% by weight maximizes biodegradability while maintaining mechanical integrity and to overcome the inherent ferromagnetic behaviour of the Fe; however, higher concentrations can lead to decreased corrosion rates due to passive layer formation (Schinhammer et al. 2013a, b). The addition of Mn alters the microstructure of the alloy, promoting the formation of galvanic cells that further accelerate degradation through localized corrosion mechanisms. Consequently, Fe–Mn alloys exhibit corrosion rates significantly higher than that of pure iron, with studies reporting rates up to 1.76 mm/year for certain compositions, thereby enhancing their effectiveness as biodegradable materials in medical applications.

Hermawan et al. (2007, 2008) conducted a pioneering study that introduced the Fe-35Mn alloy (iron with 35 wt% manganese), highlighting its potential as a biomaterial. The alloy was noted for its antiferromagnetic properties, which reduced magnetic susceptibility and made it compatible with MRI, an improvement over the highly ferromagnetic nature of pure iron. Additionally, the alloy exhibited favorable corrosion characteristics. The difference in standard electrode potentials between Fe and Mn leads to the formation of a less noble Fe–Mn solid solution, which degrades more rapidly than Fe alone. Analysis of the microstructure, corrosion resistance, magnetic properties, and toxicological aspects of the Fe–Mn alloy suggests that manganese can help improve the degradation rate.

Hermawan et al. (2010a, b, 2010c) found that adding Mn (20–35 wt.%) to Fe increased the corrosion rate, but it declined when Mn exceeded 30 wt.%. Various post processing such as rolling and heat treatments also done of Fe–Mn alloys. Figure 4.2 show the microstrure of Fe–Mn alloys before and after immersion test. Fe–Mn alloys showed minimal inhibition of 3T3 fibroblast cells compared to pure Mn. A 35 wt.% Mn alloy had a higher degradation rate (1.76 mmpy) than pure Fe (0.14 mmpy) (Hermawan et al. 2008). Chou et al. (2013) reported similar results for 3D-printed Fe-30Mn alloys.

Čapek et al. (2016a) explored the development of a Fe-30Mn alloy, revealing a corrosion rate 20 times higher than that of pure iron in potentiodynamic polarization (PDP) tests. However, in immersion tests using simulated body fluid (SBF), a reduced degradation rate was observed, attributed to the formation of a passive layer.

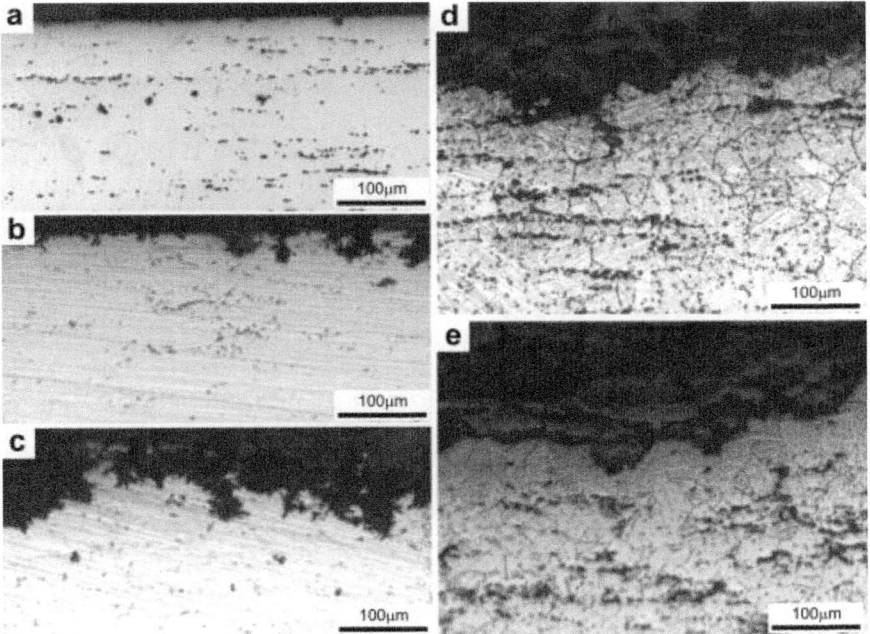

Fig. 4.2 Cross-sectional profile of polished Fe–Mn specimens: **a** before and **b, c** after 1 week and 3 months of degradation test respectively, and (d and e) etched Fe25Mn and Fe35Mn specimens after 3 months of degradation test respectively (etchant: Nital 2%). Reprinted with permission of Elsevier from Hermawan et al. (2010c)

Traverson et al. (2018) inserted the cold-drawn Fe-30Mn alloy into the bones of Sprague–Dawley rats to examine its in vivo behavior. After six months, partial resorption occurred, with increased bone cell integration compared to conventional SS316L, and no inflammatory reactions were noted. While the alloy was deemed biocompatible, it is important to acknowledge the potential neurotoxic effects of high manganese concentrations (Crossgrove and Zheng 2004; Aschner et al. 2007). Drynda et al. (2015) also investigated Fe–Mn alloys with lower manganese contents (0.5 to 6.9 wt.%), showing promising degradation rates in vitro. However, during in vivo studies, significant degradation was limited due to the formation of a phosphate passivation film.

Recently more studies on Fe–Mn alloys were done with different various powder metallurgy, additive manufacturing rout for enhanced biomineralization and biodegradtion (Sahu et al. 2024; Godec et al. 2024; Ajami et al. 2024). Different surface modification techniques also adapted on Fe–Mn system for better bioactivity (Elborolosy et al. 2023).

4.2.2 Fe–Mn-X Alloy System

Inorder to enhance the degradation and biological performance of Fe–Mn system, a combination of other alloying elements such as Pd, Cu, Ag, Ca, Mg, W and C along with Mn as the principal alloying element was also explored by researchers. This elements are capable of modifying the microstructure and there by altering the properties in an effective ways. According to Schinhammer et al. (2010), adding a small amount of Pd to Fe-10Mn increased the degradation rate by four times due to the creation of a solid solution and galvanic interactions between the Fe matrix and Pd-rich phases. In a later study, they examined the Fe-21Mn alloy system with carbon and Pd additions (Fe-21Mn-0.7C, Fe-21Mn-0.7C-1Pd), finding that both alloys exhibited a notable reduction in polarization resistance (by 102 $\Omega \cdot cm^2$), suggesting accelerated degradation (Schinhammer et al. 2013a, b). Hong et al. (2016) tested the effects of Ca and Mg additions on Fe-35Mn, finding higher corrosion current densities for Fe-35Mn-1Ca (2.12), Fe-35Mn-2Ca (6.36), Fe-35Mn-1 Mg (5.89), and Fe-35Mn-2 Mg (9.16 $\mu A \cdot cm^2$) compared to Fe-35Mn (1.00 $\mu A \cdot cm^2$). Silicon has also shown promise, with Liu et al. (2011) reporting that 1 wt.% Si doubled the corrosion current density of Fe-30Mn. Xu et al. (2015a) created Fe-28Mn alloys with up to 8% Si, noting that Fe-28Mn-6Si degraded 80% faster than Fe–Mn due to duplex phases and localized pitting. Drevet et al. (2018) demonstrated that adding 5% Si increased the degradation rate of Fe-30Mn to 0.80 mmpy. Trincă et al. (2021) reported that Ca-containing FeMnSi alloys had lower corrosion resistance and promoted osteoinduction and osteoconduction in rabbits.

Mandal et al. (2019) investigated Fe–Mn-Cu alloys (x = 0–10 wt.% Cu), observing sixfold higher degradation rates and strong antimicrobial effects, with no impact on cytocompatibility The effect of adding Cu into Fe matrix on hardness and corrosion behaviour is given in Fig. 4.3. Hufenbach et al. (2017) found that adding 0.025 wt.%

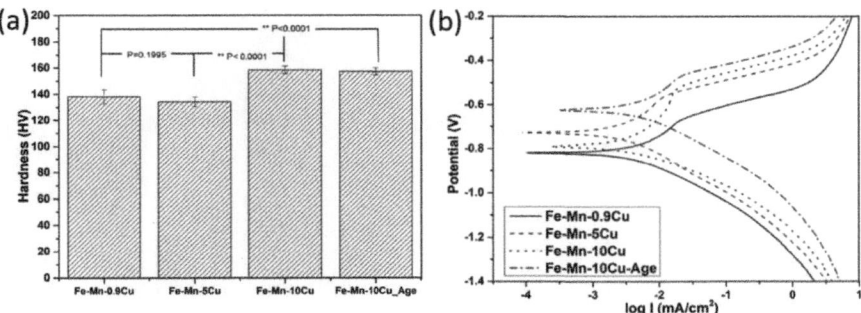

Fig. 4.3 **a** Vickers Hardness of Fe–Mn–xCu (x = 0.9, 5 and 10 wt.%) alloys and **b** potentiodynamic polarization curves measured in Hank's salt solution. Reprinted with permission of Elsevier from Mandal et al. (2019)

S to Fe-30Mn-1C increased degradation by 10% due to MnS formation, with no cytotoxic effects on L929 cells. Paul et al. (2024) investigated the effects of alloy composition on the corrosion behavior and antibacterial properties of biodegradable FeMnC and FeMnC(Cu) alloys. The addition of Cu significantly influenced degradation, as shown by immersion studies that revealed increased Fe and Mn ion release and a more porous degradation layer. However, short-term electrochemical tests did not confirm Cu's effect, suggesting the need for time-dependent studies to further investigate corrosion mechanisms. The study also compared the antibacterial properties of these alloys to 316L stainless steel. FeMnC exhibited strong antibacterial activity against S. aureus, P. aeruginosa, and E. coli, likely due to reactive oxygen species (ROS) generated during corrosion. Cu addition enhanced the antibacterial effect only for P. aeruginosa, a key pathogen in coronary stent infections, suggesting FeMnCCu could be a promising material for temporary stents.

Kraus et al. (2014) studied Fe-based alloys (Fe-10Mn-1Pd and Fe-21Mn-0.7C-1Pd) implanted in the femoral bone of Sprague–Dawley rats. Mild edema occurred post-surgery for 1–2 days. Histology revealed mostly Fe3 + and fewer Fe2 + ions near the implants, with no inflammation or tissue damage. Fântânariu et al. (2015) found that subcutaneous Fe–Mn-Si implants were more biocompatible than tibial ones but degraded slowly. Porous Fe–Mn-Si alloys with less than 4 wt.% Si degraded faster due to their structure (Xu et al. 2015b).

Fiocchi et al. (2021) investigated addition of Si into the Fe–Mn. The Fe-30Mn-5Si alloy shows strong potential for biodegradable implant applications, offering several advantages over the widely studied Fe-30Mn alloy as shown in Fig. 4.4. The addition of Sienhances workability, microstructural uniformity, and mechanical properties. A reliable production process, involving vacuum induction melting, rolling, and heat treatment, has been established, making it suitable for real-world applications. Degradation tests in simulated physiological conditions indicate that Si addition initially reduces corrosion but increases the overall degradation rate over time.

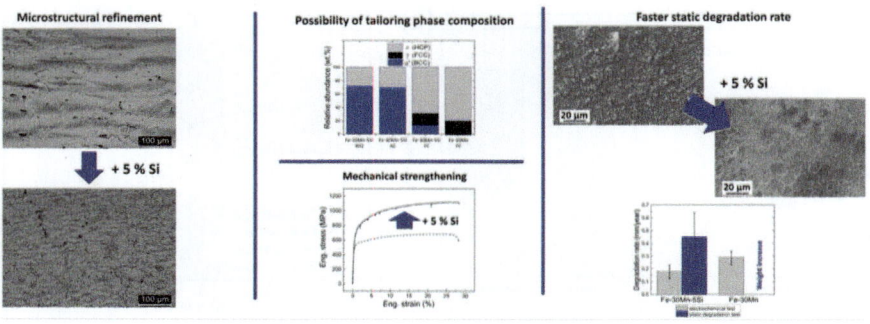

Fig. 4.4 Effect of Si addition to Fe–Mn alloy. Reprinted with permission of Elsevier from Fiocchi et al. (2021)

Elborolosy et al (2023) highlights the significance of alloying elements such as Co, W, and Cu, positioning them as valuable components in the development of biodegradable Fe. Novel nanostructured biodegradable metal alloys such as Fe–Mn–Cu, Fe–Mn–W, and Fe–Mn–Co have shown promising biocompatibility, particularly on oral epithelial cell lines. These alloys were observed to enhance cell proliferation in a time-dependent manner, with Fe–Mn–Co exhibiting the highest level of biocompatibility. Additionally, these alloys demonstrated potential anti-cancer activity, notably against the MG-63 osteosarcoma cell line, where Fe–Mn–Cu was particularly effective. Recent studies have increasingly focused on Fe–Mn-X alloys due to their distinctive properties, such as enhanced degradation rates and low magnetic susceptibility.

4.2.3 Fe–X Alloy System

Apart form Mn, other elements also used for the developing Fe based implants. In most cases, either powder metallurgy or additive manufacturing techniques were used to produce these alloys. Ag, Pt, Wegener et al. (2011) developed and and tested various alloys, including Fe–C, Fe–0.6P, Fe–1.6P, Fe–B, and Fe–Ag. The results indicated that carbon-containing alloys exhibited the highest corrosion rates, while samples with phosphorus, silver, and boron showed only a slight increase in degradation. Pure iron had the lowest rate of corrosion. Additionally, Čapek's et al. (2016b) produced pure Fe and Fe alloys (Pd, Ag, and C) using powder metallurgy. Limited diffusion occurred between Fe and Pd or C during sintering thus Pd and C significantly enhanced the corrosion rate of Fe in immersion tests, while Ag decreased the corrosion rate. Overall, Pd and C show promise for improving the degradation of Fe-based biodegradable materials.

Wang et al. (2017b) explored how Ga, along with B and Ta, influences the degradation behavior of Fe. They examined Fe-19 Ga, (Fe-19 Ga)-2B, and (Fe-19 Ga)-0.5(TaC) alloys. The inclusion of Ga in Fe raised the corrosion rate to 0.48 mmpy, with B further increasing it to 0.63 mmpy, while Ta exhibited a relatively lower corrosion rate of 0.33 mmpy. Notably, all these alloys showed higher corrosion rates compared to pure Fe (0.13 mmpy). Surface analysis after a 28-day immersion in SBF revealed that Fe-19 Ga experienced the most significant surface loss. Additionally, cell culture tests indicated that MC3T3-E1 cells adhered and proliferated well on Fe-Ga alloy surfaces.

4.3   Microstructure Modification

Incorporating secondary phases into the Fe matrix is another strategy for accelerating the degradation rate of Fe-based composites for biodegradable applications. These secondary phases, which can include noble elements Pt, Au, Ag and Pd, or even bioceramic reinforcements, act as cathodic sites within the predominantly anodic Fe matrix. By forming micro-galvanic couples, these cathodes create localized electrochemical environments that significantly reduce the corrosion potential of the Fe matrix while simultaneously increasing the corrosion current. This enhanced electrochemical activity leads to a more rapid dissolution of the Fe, thus facilitating a controlled and accelerated degradation process. The presence of these secondary phases not only promotes effective biodegradation but also allows for better tunability of the alloy's mechanical properties, bioactivity and biocompatibility, ensuring that the composite can meet specific requirements for temporary implants while minimizing adverse effects on surrounding tissues.

4.3.1   Microstructure Modification by Noble Elements

Studies by Huang et al. (2014, 2016a) explored the addition of noble metals like Au, Pt, Pd, and Ag as secondary phases to enhance degradation. These elements form fine, uniformly distributed intermetallic phases, promoting galvanic corrosion by providing more active sites within the iron matrix (Zheng et al. 2014).

Pd is used to enhance the biodegradability of iron due to its higher nobility (+0.99 V vs. SHE) and ability to stabilize iron in its non-magnetic austenite state, which is ideal for implant applications. Pd is miscible with Fe at high temperatures and can be precipitated within the Fe matrix through proper heat treatment. Studies by Schinhammer et al. (2010, 2012, 2013a, b) demonstrated that adding 1 wt.% Pd to the Fe–Mn system doubled the degradation rate in a 28-day immersion test in SBF, driven by the creation of micro galvanic cells due to uniformly distributed Pd-rich phases. The precipitate also strengthens the alloy by reducing the Zener drag effect at the grain boundaries. Ag is another noble metal used to increase Fe-based implants' degradation rates due to its high electrochemical potential (+0.800 vs. SHE), biocompatibility, and antibacterial properties. Research has shown that adding 2 wt.% of Ag and Pd to Fe-based alloys boosts degradation rates without affecting cytocompatibility, making them safe for biomedical applications as long as ion release remains within tolerance limits (Čapek et al. 2016b).

Other noble metals such as Pt and Au are employed to accelerate the degradation of Fe. Pt (+1.18 V vs SHE) and Au (+1.69 V vs SHE) have a high electrochemical potential and are biocompatible, making them an ideal secondary phase in Fe matrix for BMs application (Geurtsen 2002; Nouri and Wen 2021; Rabeeh et al. 2023). Huang et al. (2014) demonstrated that alloying iron with 5 wt.% of Pd and Pt significantly enhances the degradation rate, particularly in Fe-Pt composites. In static immersion tests, the degradation rate increased by 50% for Fe-Pd and 100% for Fe-Pt, attributed to the finely dispersed Pd and Pt phases forming micro-galvanic couplings with the Fe matrix. These alloys showed no cytotoxicity towards L-929 and ECV304 cells. Similar results were observed for Fe-Au and Fe-Ag composites with 2, 5, and 10 wt.% Au or Ag in immersion tests, also showing no cytotoxic effects (Huang et al. 2016a, b, c). Sharipova et al. (2019) developed Fe-Ag nanocomposites, which exhibited a 4 to 20-fold increase in degradation rates due to the formation of numerous nano-galvanic cells, far surpassing their micro-grain counterparts. This demonstrates the potential of noble metal alloying in enhancing the degradation and biocompatibility of iron-based implants.

Recently Rabeeh et al. (2023) developed Fe-Au composites with minimal content, via powder metallurgy, demonstrate promising results for biodegradable implants. The addition of Au enhances the degradation rate of Fe by threefold in physiological environments, improving interfacial properties and cell viability. The study showed that Fe-nAu composites exhibited greater viability for L929 cells, with enhanced cell attachment and proliferation as shown in Fig. 4.5. After 28 days of immersion, the Au-incorporated samples degraded at a rate of 1.29 mm/year, compared to 0.36 mm/year for pure Fe. The major reason for this higher degradation rate is due to the galvanic coupling between the Fe and Au in the matrix as shown in Fig. 4.6.

4.3.2 Microstructure Modification by Bioceramics

For effective tissue integration, implants require bioactive nature that support osteo-conductivity and encourage bone tissue growth and natural apatite formation. Incorporating bioactive materials like calcium phosphate, calcium silicate, and akermanite into the Fe matrix can enhance both mechanical properties and bioactivity. It is reported that dispersion of soluble bioceramics in Fe matrix can improve the biodegradation rate (Ulum et al. 2014; Montufar et al. 2016; Wang et al. 2017a; Shuai et al. 2019; Gao et al. 2020, Rabeeh et al. 2024a).

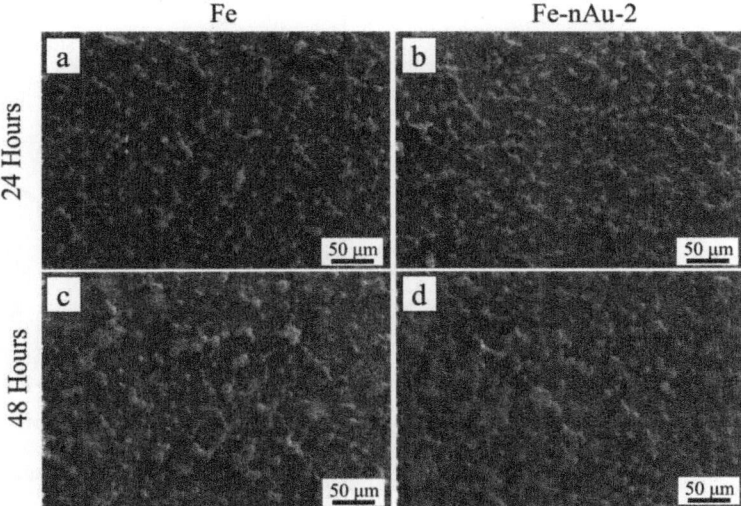

Fig. 4.5 SEM imaging of the surface of the sample with adhered L929 cells after cell fixation. Reprinted with permission of American Chemical Society from Rabeeh et al. (2023)

4.3.2.1 Calcium Phosphate Based Bioceramics

Calcium phosphate (CaP) based biocemamics such as hydroxyapatite (HA), trical-cium phosphate (TCP), biphasic calcium phosphate (BCP) are known for their excellent biocompatibility and osteoconductive properties, making them ideal for enhancing the performance of Fe matrices. When incorporated into the Fe matrix, calcium phosphates not only improve the mechanical properties but also significantly accelerate the degradation rate of the composite. For instance, studies have shown that adding calcium phosphate can increase the degradation rate by several times compared to pure iron, facilitating a more controlled release of ions that promote cell proliferation and tissue integration (Ulum et al. 2014; Reindl et al. 2014; Rabeeh and Hanas 2022a, b; Rabeeh et al. 2024a, b; Chebodaeva et al. 2024; Bulutsuz et al. 2024). Additionally, the presence of calcium phosphate enhances bioactivity, allowing for better interaction with surrounding biological tissues and ultimately supporting effective healing processes in temporary implant applications.

Ulum et al. (2014) reported that the incorporation of 5 wt.% of HA)/5 wt.% TCP/ 5 wt.% BCP- 40wt.% HA and 60wt.% TCP to Fe matrix to achieve and enhanced the degradation rate due to the multiphase structure as shown in Fig. 4.7. The composite showed a substantial increase in its degradation rate over pure Fe during in vitro immersion testing. When tested in SBF for 14 days, the incorporation of HA, TCP, and BCP into the Fe matrix led to a 2, 5, and threefold enhancement in the degradation rate, respectively. Furthermore, the bioceramic components enhanced biocompatibility by 20% compared to pure Fe. This is due to the.

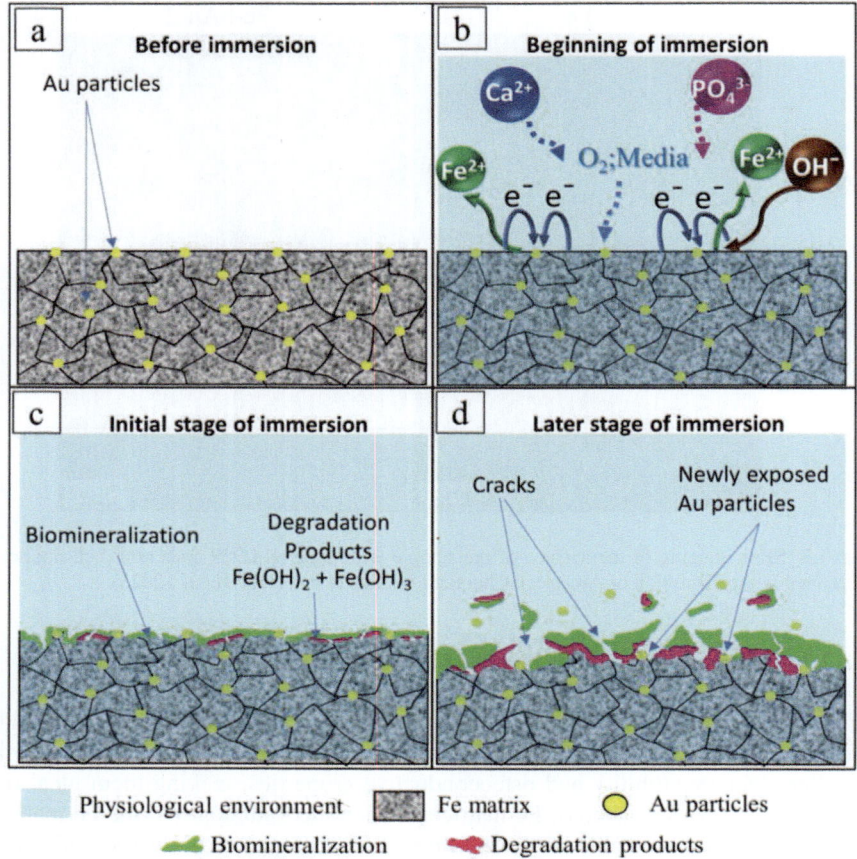

Fig. 4.6 Degradation mechanism of Fe-nAu in the physiological environment. Reprinted with permission of American Chemical Society from Rabeeh et al. (2023)

In a study by Reindl et al. (2014), the influence of incorporating varying volume percentages (30, 40, and 50%) of β-tricalcium phosphate (β-TCP) into a pure iron (Fe) matrix on degradation rates was investigated through an extended in vitro immersion test conducted in a 0.9% NaCl solution. Results after 56 days revealed that all samples experienced an increase in degradation rate, with the composite containing 40 vol% β-TCP showing a notable 28% rise, highlighting the significant impact of this specific β-TCP concentration on enhancing degradation.

Tripathi and Pandey (2024) used an innovative fabrication technique that integrates 3D printing via stereolithography, pressureless microwave sintering, and casting to develop topologically ordered, functionally graded composite (TOFGC) biodegradable implants. This adaptive method enables diverse mechanical and degradation profiles by modifying the unit cell structure and zinc infiltration in Fe-HA

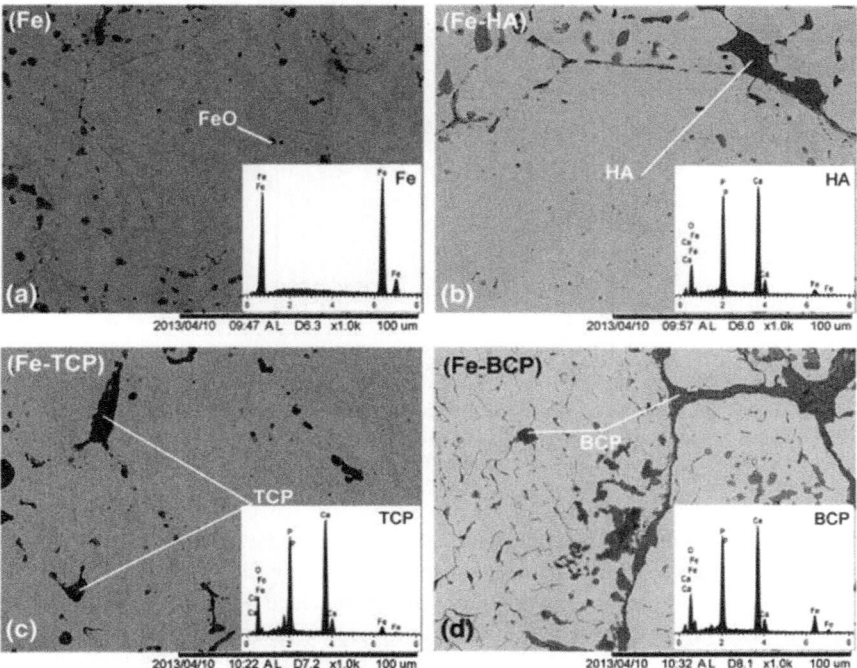

Fig. 4.7 SEM images of the the Fe-matrix composite showing the bioceramic phases. Reprinted with permission of Elsevier from Ulum et al. (2014)

scaffolds. It ensures implant safety for bone tissue engineering by preventing mold material contamination and allows for customizable mechanical properties to suit various clinical needs. The density, porosity, compressive yield strength (CYS), and modulus of elasticity of the fabricated implants span a wide range—1.95–5.36 g/cm³, 28.37–73.99%, 17.62–102.32 MPa, and 186.12–245.20 MPa, respectively. Notably, CYS and Young's modulus increase with higher zinc infiltration, and the electrochemical and static immersion tests confirm that zinc content significantly influences the degradation properties of the TOFGC biomaterial. Corrosion rates range from 1.68 mm/year to 4.33 mm/year, with the highest observed in zinc-infused Fe-HA scaffolds. Overall, this technique offers a promising pathway for creating bone implants with optimized and customizable mechanical and degradation characteristics that outperform traditional irregular porous iron scaffolds.

In recent study, Rabeeh et al. (2024a, b) explained the degradation mechanism (Fig. 4.8) of Fe– nano-hydroxyapatite (nHA) composites incorporating 1.5 wt% and 3 wt% nHA were fabricated using powder metallurgy techniques to improve their degradation rates in physiological environments. The incorporation of nHA would enhance the number of defects in the Fe matrix, which also acts as active sites for the reactions and leads to the degradation of the Fe. The nHA agglomerates

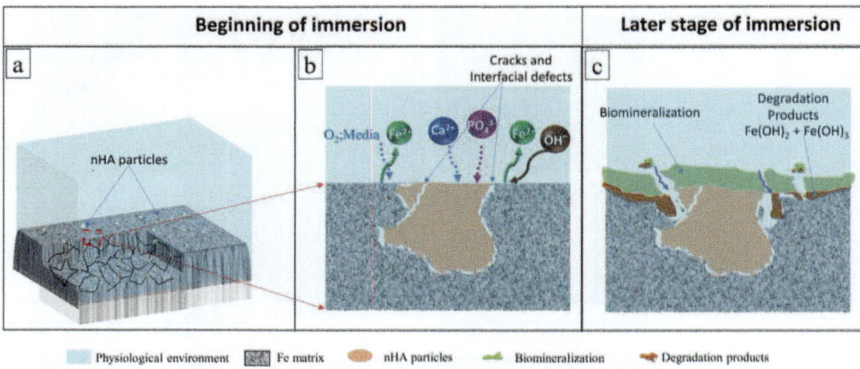

Fig. 4.8 Schematics of the mechanism of formation of biomineralization and degradation of the Fe–nHA composite sample. **a, b** Initials stage of immersion and **c** latter stage of immersion. Reprinted with permission of Springer Nature from Rabeeh et al. (2024a, b)

contain micro-voids and interface with the surrounding Fe matrix contains porosity and micro- cracks due the shrinkage at interface during the sintering process. The presence of these pores and microcracks at the interface between Fe and nHA can serve as pathways for the entry of medium into the Fe matrix. This can increase probability of localized and crevice corrosion, in addition to the more typically seen uniform corrosion. Notably, the addition of 3% nHA resulted in a remarkable five-fold increase in the degradation rate of Fe. Beyond enhancing degradation, nHA integration also improved the bioactivity and wettability of the Fe matrix, leading to enhanced biocompatibility. In vitro cytocompatibility assessments revealed that the Fe–nHA composite samples demonstrated increased viability and proliferation of L-929 cells. After 28 days of immersion, the samples containing 3% nHA exhibited a degradation rate of 1.3 mmpy, significantly higher than the 0.35 mmpy observed for pure Fe.

4.3.2.2 Silicate Based Bioceramics

Silicate ($-SiO_4$)-based bioceramics are also used for enhancing the properties of Fe-based biodegradable implants. These bioceramics, known for their excellent bioactivity, can be incorporated into Fe matrices to improve osteoconductivity and promote bone regeneration. When combined with Fe, silicate enhances the mechanical properties of the composite while providing a favorable environment for cell adhesion and tissue integration. The presence of silicate facilitates the release of bioactive ions that stimulate biomineralization and osteogenesis, thereby accelerating the healing process.

Wang et al. (2017a) developed an Fe-based bioceramic composite incorporating a substantial quantity (20–40 wt.%) of calcium silicate (Ca_2SiO_4) as a secondary phase. The fine dispersion of Ca_2SiO_4 within the Fe matrix resulted in compressive and bending strengths comparable to human bone while significantly enhancing degradation rates in simulated body fluid (SBF) over a 7-day period. Notably, adding 20 wt.% Ca_2SiO_4 to iron tripled the degradation rate, and increasing the content to 40 wt.% led to an eightfold increase. Additionally, the composite with 20 wt.% Ca_2SiO_4 showed superior capability in supporting human bone marrow stromal cell (hBMSC) proliferation compared to pure iron.

Bredigite (BR) is another silicate bioceramics with a nominal composition of $Ca_7MgSi_4O_{16}$. Shuai et al (2016) successfully fabricated an Fe/BR composite using laser additive manufacturing technology, achieving a high densification rate and a uniform distribution of BR within the Fe matrix. The Fe/5.0BR composite exhibited significant improvements in mechanical properties, with increases of 79.8% in compressive yield strength, 52.7% in ultimate strength, and 25.5% in hardness. Electrochemical and immersion tests revealed an accelerated corrosion rate in the composite, primarily due to local pitting corrosion from BR's rapid dissolution. Furthermore, BR enhanced cellular proliferation and differentiation, likely due to the composite's improved bioactivity and nutrient element release. Overall, Fe/BR shows promise as a bone repair material, combining robust mechanical properties, a suitable degradation rate, and favorable biocompatibility.

4.3.3 Microstructure Modification by Other Particles

Apart from noble metals and biocermaics, mateirals like carbon nanotubes (CNT), graphene oxides (GO), iron oxide (Fe_2O_3) and magnesium silicide (Mg_2Si) are also used for modifying the microstructure of Fe matrix thereby enhancing the degradation behaviour.

Cheng and Zheng (2013) investigated the effects of adding carbon nanotubes (CNT) to Fe matrix, finding that CNT additions (0.5 and 1 wt.%) accelerated corrosion by thirteen times in electrochemical tests and nearly doubled degradation in immersion tests. The composites displayed satisfactory cytocompatibility and hemocompatibility. In a follow-up study, Cheng et al. (2014) explored the effects of incorporating Fe_2O_3 into Fe for degradable implant use across various concentrations (2, 5, 10, and 50 wt.%). At lower Fe_2O_3 concentrations (2 and 5 wt.%), a new FeO phase appeared, with all composites exhibiting increased degradation rates, particularly the 5% Fe_2O_3 composition. Biocompatibility testing with cell lines L929, VSMC, and ECV304 confirmed the biocompatibility of all Fe-Fe_2O_3 composites. Oriňáková et al. (2013a) observed that adding 0.5 wt.% CNT to Fe-based scaffolds reduced the degradation rate twofold in Hank's solution over eight weeks, while the same amount of Mg doubled the degradation rate. Similarly, Sikora-Jasinska et al. (2019) reported that a 1 wt.% Mg_2Si addition to Fe also doubled its degradation rate, with a unique corrosion mechanism in Fe-Mg2Si composites in modified Hank's solution due to preferential Mg dissolution and Fe pitting at the matrix-reinforcement interface.

In a study by Zhao et al. (2020), the influence of graphene oxide (GO) on iron-based composites was examined by fabricating Fe-xGO (where x varies from 0.4 wt.% to 1.6 wt.%) with uniformly distributed GO nanoparticles as a secondary phase. Their electrochemical analyses revealed that with increased GO content, the corrosion potential (Ecorr) shifted negatively, suggesting an accelerated degradation rate. Similarly, immersion tests indicated that iron ion release was about 20% higher than that of pure iron, indicating a more rapid degradation of Fe-xGO composites, likely due to micro-galvanic coupling between the GO and the Fe matrix.

4.4 Surface Modification

Surface modification is a common approach for tailoring the bioactivity, biocompatibility and degradation of BMs. Treatments on the metal surfaces can help in tailoring the bioactivity, resulting in improved osteointegration and hemocompatibility (Gao et al. 2017; Hanas et al. 2018; Ansari 2019; Al-Amin et al. 2020; Oriňaková et al. 2020; Rahim et al. 2021). Various techniques are employed to tailor the implant surfaces are given in Fig. 4.9.

4.4.1 Coating

Coating is a surface modification strategy to enhance the performance of BMs and biocompatibility in medical applications. Various type of coatings such as polymeric, noble metal coating and laser treatments are employed onto the implant surface. These coatings improve osseointegration by promoting cell adhesion and proliferation while also providing a protective barrier that enhances corrosion resistance and

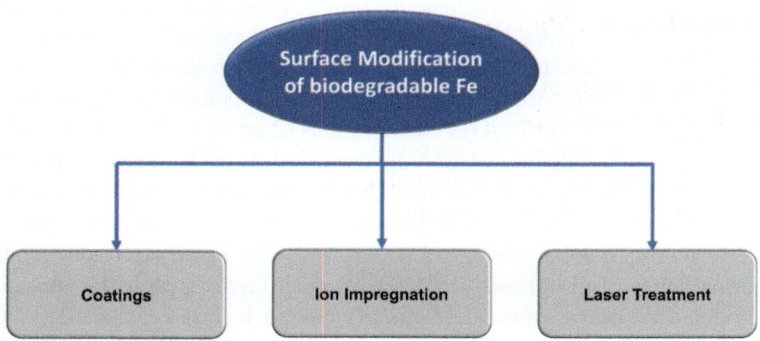

Fig. 4.9 Classification of surface modifications

reduces the release of metallic ions into surrounding tissues especially during the intial period of implantation.

4.4.1.1 Polymer Coating

Biodegradable polymer coatings are increasingly utilized on iron (Fe) implants to enhance their biocompatibility and control degradation rates, providing a protective barrier that promotes osseointegration while allowing for the gradual release of bioactive substances. In a study conducted by Yusop et al. (2015), they explored the impact of poly(lactic-co-glycolic acid) (PLGA) coatings on porous iron (Fe) structures. By employing a vacuum infiltration technique, they created dense PLGA-filled porous Fe, and for a less dense coating, they utilized a dip-coating method. During a four-week immersion test in phosphate-buffered saline (PBS), the dense PLGA-filled Fe demonstrated a substantial degradation rate of 6.42 mmpy, outperforming both the low-density PLGA-filled and uncoated porous Fe, which showed degradation rates of 0.76 and 0.33 mmpy, respectively. The accelerated degradation in the PLGA-coated samples was primarily attributed to the hydrolytic breakdown of the PLGA, which resulted in a localized decrease in pH, aiding in the dissolution of degradation products and promoting further degradation. Despite this enhanced degradation rate, the PLGA coating did not adversely affect the cytocompatibility of human fibroblast cells.

Similarly, Haverová et al. (2018) examined the effect of poly-ethylene glycol (PEG) coating on Fe foam, noting a shift in corrosion potential toward more negative values, which increased the corrosion rate to between 0.53 and 0.70 mmpy—considerably higher than uncoated Fe. Following a 12-week immersion in simulated body fluid (SBF), the PEG-coated samples exhibited almost double the weight loss of uncoated Fe, likely due to the intimate contact between the hydrophilic PEG layer and the Fe surface. Oriňaková et al. (2019) assessed the biocompatibility of PEG-coated Fe foams, reporting over 90% viability in human dermal fibroblast (HDFa) cells, with cell growth 20–50% higher than with pure Fe extract.

Qi et al. (2019) highlighted the effectiveness of metal-polymer composite coatings, such as poly(methyl methacrylate) (PMMA) and polylactic acid (PLA), in controlling Fe degradation under biomimetic conditions (Fig. 4.10). PLA-coated Fe exhibited a corrosion current density nearly three times that of uncoated or PMMA-coated Fe, likely due to the hydrolysis of PLA, which produces carboxyl groups, influencing H + and lactate ion activity on Fe degradation. PLA's hydrolysis was found to help prevent passive layer deposition, thereby elevating local pH and increasing Fe degradation. Hrubovčáková et al. (2017) corroborated these findings, showing faster degradation in PLA-coated Fe foams than in uncoated counterparts. Additionally, Gorejová et al. (2020) indicated that varying polymer concentration offers an effective approach for tuning degradation rates in biomedical applications.

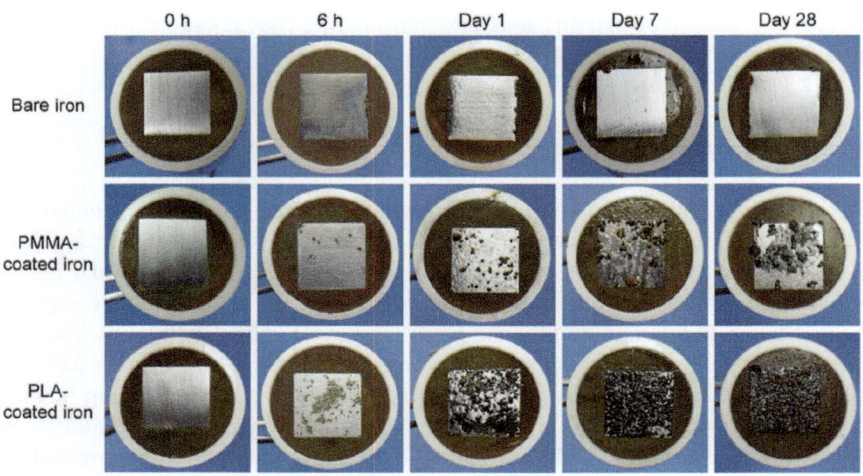

Fig. 4.10 Degradation morphologies of Fe with and without polymer coatings after immersion in Hank's solution. (Reprinted with permission of Springer Nature from Rabeeh and Hanas 2022a, b)

4.4.1.2 Noble Metal Coating/patterning

Coating or pattering noble metals onto Fe-based biomaterials has been shown to enhance their degradation rates. For instance, Cheng et al. (2015) demonstrated that a vacuum-sputtered, micro-patterned array of gold (Au) on iron surfaces accelerates degradation. They examined two distinct Au array sizes (200×200 μm^2 and 50×50 μm^2) on pure iron and observed significantly increased corrosion rates of 2.338 and 3.174 $g \cdot m^{-2} \cdot d^{-1}$, respectively, compared to the unmodified Fe corrosion rate of 0.617 $g \cdot m^{-2} \cdot d^{-1}$. This increase was attributed to the formation of a galvanic cell between the Au discs and Fe, promoting a uniform corrosion pattern.

Similarly, Huang and Zheng (2016) developed a patterned array of platinum (Pt) discs on iron (Fig. 4.11), which also notably enhanced the degradation rate in both electrochemical and immersion tests, showing nearly triple the degradation rate of uncoated Fe. In terms of biocompatibility, these modified Fe specimens were found non-toxic to EA.hy926 endothelial cells but effectively inhibited the proliferation of vascular smooth muscle cells (VSMCs).

Rabeeh and Hanas (2022a, b) investigated the gold sputtering on porous Fe to enhance degradation rates in physiological environments. Electrochemical corrosion tests and static immersion studies demonstrated that both gold sputtering and porosity synergistically accelerated iron's degradation process. The degradation mechanism of such surface pattering or coating is because of the formation of galvanic coupling between the noble metal and Fe surface (Fig. 4.12). The incorporation of gold at the sample interface was shown to promote cell viability, adhesion, and proliferation on the sample surfaces. However, the degradation rate reduction observed due to the limited presence of gold in the sample's bulk material. Thus this kind of noble metal

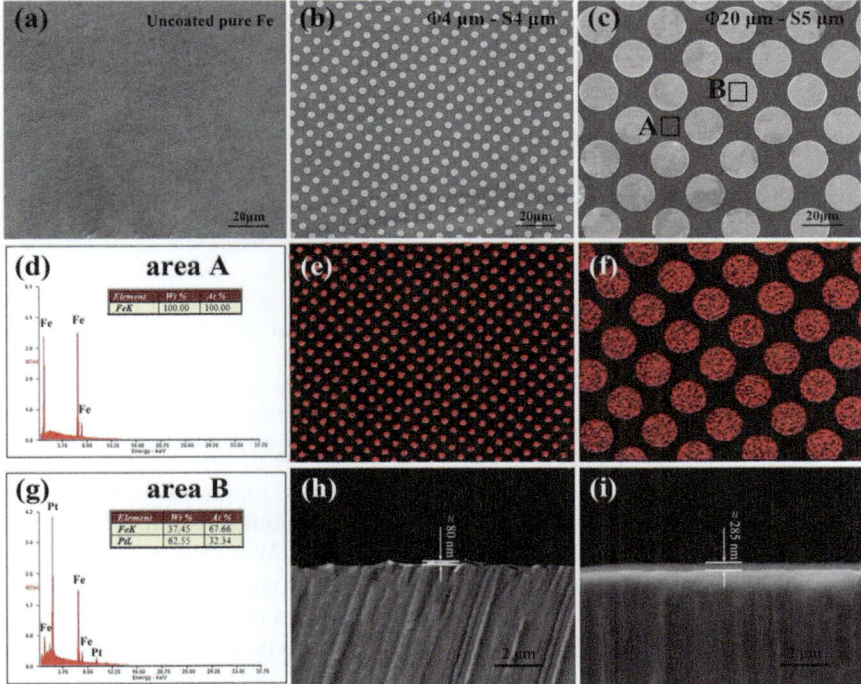

Fig. 4.11 Microstructure of Pt discs patterned pure iron: **a** uncoated pure iron, **b** Φ4 μm × S4 μm and **c** Φ20 μm × S5 μm Pt discs patterned pure iron, **d** and **g** are energy spectrum analysis related to area A and B respectively, **e** and **f** are energy spectrum plane scanning analysis of Pt, **h** and **i** are the cross sections of Φ4 μm × S4 μm and Φ20 μm × S5 μm patterned pure iron, respectively. Reprinted from Huang and Zheng (2016) under CC BY 4.0

suface patterning can be used only for certain implant application requiring a high surface to volume ratio, such as stents, bone cages, thin plates, and suture lines.

4.4.1.3 Other Coatings

Apart from polymeric and noble metal coating other type of coating such as electrode-position, electrophoretic deposition, nitriding are also used for modifying the surface of Fe materials. In a study by Adhilakshmi et al. (2020), the authors demonstrated that the cathodic electrodeposition of a zinc–zinc phosphate–calcium phosphate composite coating on pure iron represents a promising method to enhance the bioac-tivity and stability of implant surfaces during the early stages of implantation. Their investigation revealed that the resulting morphology of the coating featured plate-like crystals with multi-directional growth and fine pores. Notably, in vitro immersion studies in simulated body fluid (SBF) indicated that this bioactive composite surface

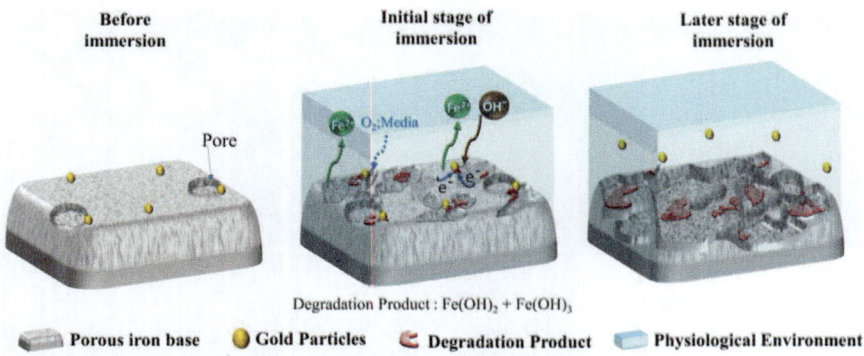

promoted the development of flower-like apatite crystals. Additionally, cytocompatibility assessments showed that the coating exhibited a commendable level of biocompatibility and significantly improved cell proliferation. Wen et al. (2013) explored the enhancement of iron foam by applying a calcium phosphate/chitosan coating through electrophoretic deposition. This modification resulted in improved degradation performance when the coated iron foam was immersed in phosphate-buffered saline (PBS) and simulated body fluid (SBF).

Huang et al. (2020) employed a spin coating technique to apply fibrillar Type I collagen onto the surface of Fe-30Mn. This innovative approach was aimed at enhancing the cell compatibility of the material. The results from their experiments indicated that the collagen-coated surface significantly improved both osteointegration and cytocompatibility of the implant material, showcasing the potential benefits of this modification for biomedical applications.

Furthermore, Chen et al. (2008) highlighted the corrosion resistance of a surface-transformed compound layer composed of two iron nitrides in a 0.9% NaCl solution. These protective films were effective in mitigating the degradation of mechanical integrity in iron-based biomaterials during the initial phase of implantation. However, contrasting findings from long-term in vitro degradation studies conducted by Feng et al. (2013) and Lin et al. (2016) indicated that the nitriding treatment on the iron surface significantly accelerated the degradation rate over time.

4.4.2   Ion Impregnation

Ion impregnation is an effective surface modification technique for enhancing the properties of biodegradable metallic implants. This method involves the incorporation of ions, such as Ag, zinc or calcium, into the surface layer of the implant material through processes like ion implantation or metal vapor vacuum arc deposition (Salama et al. 2022). By embedding these ions, the surface characteristics of the Fe matrix can be significantly tailor the degradtion and biocompatibility. The implanted ions can create micro-galvanic couples that accelerate degradation rates, which is beneficial for temporary implants designed to dissolve after fulfilling their function in the body. Additionally, ion impregnation can modify the surface energy and roughness, promoting better cell adhesion and proliferation, thereby improving the overall integration of the implant with surrounding tissues.

Huang et al. (2016b) enhanced the degradation properties of pure iron by introducing silver (Ag) ions into its surface using the metal vapor vacuum arc (MEVVA) technique. This method created a surface layer approximately 60 nm thick composed of Ag and Ag_2O, with Ag diffusing into the iron subsurface. These Ag-based surface modifications accelerated the iron's degradation rate through galvanic corrosion, as shown in electrochemical and immersion tests. The corrosion rate notably increased during the initial immersion period, roughly doubling due to Ag implantation. However, after 15 days, the degradation rate stabilized as the Ag-rich layer eroded. Biocompatibility tests with L-929, EA.hy926, and VSMC cells showed a slight reduction in cell viability compared to pure iron, though this reduction remained within safe limits. In related work, the authors also investigated the effects of zinc (Zn) implantation on iron surfaces enhances the degradation as evidented from Fig. 4.13. (Huang et al. 2016c). Zhu et al. (2009) used similar method for Lanthanum ion implantation at a 40 kV extracted voltage to improve the surface properties and delay the degradation rate of Fe during the initial implantation period.

4.4.3 Laser Treatment

Laser-assisted surface modification is an innovative technique that utilizes focused laser beams to alter the surface characteristics of the Fe, allowing for precise control over microstructural changes and surface morphology. By melting or vaporizing specific surface layers, laser treatment can create a refined microstructure that improves mechanical strength and corrosion resistance. The rapid heating and cooling cycles involved in laser processing also enable the formation of unique surface features, such as micro-patterns, nano-pattern or porous structures, which enhance cell adhesion and proliferation.

Sun et al. (2021) investigated the effects of varying degrees of ablation on the degradable Fe–30Mn alloy, utilizing both continuous and pulsed lasers, specifically nanosecond and femtosecond lasers. The findings indicated that the nanostructures produced by femtosecond laser treatment significantly increased the surface area of the alloy, which correspondingly elevated its corrosion rate by approximately 40%. Furthermore, the researchers noted that the laser-modified surfaces of the Fe–30Mn alloy enhanced both biodegradability and biocompatibility, making them suitable for biological applications. Supporting these findings, Hočevar et al. (2017) reported

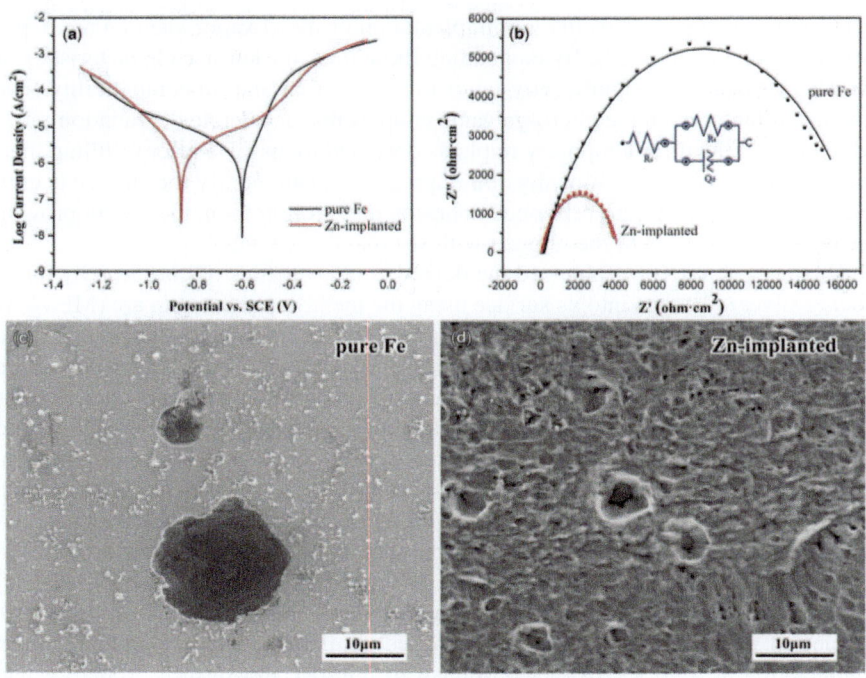

Fig. 4.13 Electrochemical measurement results: **a** Tafel curves, **b** Nyquist plots, **c** and **d** are the surface morphologies of specimens after potentiodynamic polarization. Reprinted from Huang et al. (2016c) under CC BY 4.0

that laser surface treatment of Fe–Mn alloys resulted in corrosion rates that were six times higher than those of non-treated counterparts.

Donik et al. (2018) examined the corrosion behavior of a Fe–Mn alloy with altered surface topology (Fig. 4.14) in Hank's solution using potentiodynamic polarization (PDP) and electrochemical impedance spectroscopy (EIS). They found that the polished alloy had a corrosion rate eight times higher than that of the unpolished version. Additionally, EIS results showed a significant reduction in charge transfer resistance after laser treatment, which the authors attributed to the creation of a super hydrophilic surface and increased surface area with nano-structured oxides formed during the process.

Biffi et al (2022) investigated the impact of ultrashort laser texturing processes on the surface characteristics, phase structure, and degradation behavior of a biodegradable Fe–20Mn alloy. The study revealed the adjustments in laser power and scanning speed were shown to significantly alter the average surface roughness, increasing it from approximately 0.03 μm to around 12 μm while maintaining the integrity of the bulk microstructure. The degradation behavior of the alloy was notably influenced by the laser power, with the morphology of the laser-treated surfaces affecting wettability and consequently the surface's interaction with the solution. Furthermore,

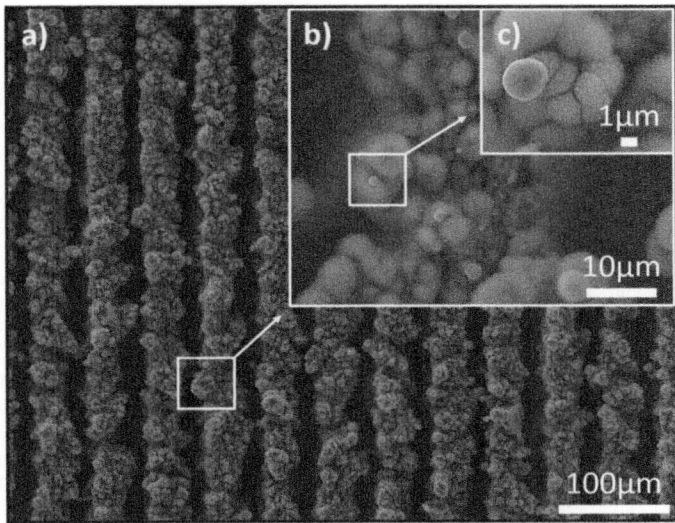

Fig. 4.14 SEM image of surface topography of Fe–Mn laser-textured sample. Reprinted with permission of Elsevier from Donik et al. (2018)

careful selection of laser power enabled the tuning of the degradation rate, leading to either an enhancement of +29% or a reduction of -31% in comparison to untreated surfaces.

References

Adhilakshmi A, Ravichandran K, Sankara Narayanan TSN (2020) Cathodic electrodeposition of zinc-zinc phosphate-calcium phosphate composite coatings on pure iron for biodegradable implant applications. New J Chem 44:6475–6489. https://doi.org/10.1039/d0nj00991a

Ajami S, Kraaneveld C, Koudstaal M, Dunaway D, Jeelani NUO, Schievano S, Bregoli C, Fiocchi J, Biffi CA, Tuissi A, Borghi A (2024) In vitro assessment of the neuro-compatibility of Fe-20Mn as a potential bioresorbable material for craniofacial surgery. Medicina 60(3):440. https://doi.org/10.3390/medicina60030440

Al-Amin M, Abdul Rani AM, Abdu Aliyu AA et al (2020) Bio-ceramic coatings adhesion and roughness of biomaterials through PM-EDM: a comprehensive review. Mater Manuf Process, 1157–1180.https://doi.org/10.1080/10426914.2020.1772483

Ansari M (2019) Bone tissue regeneration: biology, strategies and interface studies. Prog Biomater 8:223–237. https://doi.org/10.1007/S40204-019-00125-Z

Aschner M, Guilarte TR, Schneider JS, Zheng W (2007) Manganese: recent advances in understanding its transport and neurotoxicity. Toxicol Appl Pharmacol 221:131–147. https://doi.org/10.1016/j.taap.2007.03.001

Beattie JH, Avenell A (1992) Trace element nutrition and bone metabolism. Nutr Res Rev 5:167–188. https://doi.org/10.1079/nrr19920013

Biffi CA, Fiocchi J, Bregoli C et al (2022) Ultrashort laser texturing for tuning surface morphology and degradation behavior of the biodegradable Fe–20Mn alloy for temporary implants. Adv Eng Mater 24:2101496. https://doi.org/10.3390/jfb13020072

Bulutsuz GA, Chrominski W, Bazarnik P, Bruder E (2024) Development of Fe-10%(HA/β-tricalcium phosphate) composite via solid-state manufacturing route and investigation of material properties for biodegradable implant applications. Adv Eng Mater 26:2301858. https://doi.org/10.1002/adem.202301858

Čapek J, Kubásek J, Vojtěch D et al (2016a) Microstructural, mechanical, corrosion and cytotoxicity characterization of the hot forged FeMn30(wt.%) alloy. Mater Sci Eng C 58:900–908. https://doi.org/10.1016/j.msec.2015.09.049

Čapek J, Stehlíková K, Michalcová A, et al (2016b) Microstructure, mechanical and corrosion properties of biodegradable powder metallurgical Fe-2 wt.% X (X = Pd, Ag and C) alloys. Mater Chem Phys 181:501–511. https://doi.org/10.1016/j.matchemphys.2016.06.087

Chebodaeva VV, Luginin NA, Rezvanova AE, Bakina OV, Svarovskaya NV, Suliz KV, Rodkevich NG (2024) Corrosion and mechanical properties of bioresorbable composite based on Fe-Cu-hydroxyapatite powders. J Alloys Compd 1005:176209. https://doi.org/10.1016/j.jallcom.2024.176209

Chen CZ, Shi XH, Zhang PC et al (2008) The microstructure and properties of commercial pure iron modified by plasma nitriding. Solid State Ion 179:971–974. https://doi.org/10.1016/j.ssi.2008.03.019

Cheng J, Huang T, Zheng YF (2015) Relatively uniform and accelerated degradation of pure iron coated with micro-patterned Au disc arrays. Mater Sci Eng C 48:679–687. https://doi.org/10.1016/j.msec.2014.12.053

Cheng J, Zheng YF (2013) In vitro study on newly designed biodegradable Fe-X composites (X = W, CNT) prepared by spark plasma sintering. J Biomed Mater Res B Appl Biomater 101:485–497. https://doi.org/10.1002/jbm.b.32783

Chou DT, Wells D, Hong D et al (2013) Novel processing of iron-manganese alloy-based biomaterials by inkjet 3-D printing. Acta Biomater 9:8593–8603. https://doi.org/10.1016/j.actbio.2013.04.016

Crossgrove J, Zheng W (2004) Manganese toxicity upon overexposure. NMR Biomed 17:544–553

Donik Č, Kocijan A, Paulin I et al (2018) Improved biodegradability of Fe–Mn alloy after modification of surface chemistry and topography by a laser ablation. Appl Surf Sci 453:383–393. https://doi.org/10.1016/j.apsusc.2018.05.066

Drevet R, Zhukova Y, Malikova P et al (2018) Martensitic transformations and mechanical and corrosion properties of Fe-Mn-Si alloys for biodegradable medical implants. Metall Mater Trans A Phys Metall Mater Sci 49:1006–1013. https://doi.org/10.1007/s11661-017-4458-2

Elborolosy SA, Hussein LA, Mahran H, Ammar HR, Sivasankaran S, Abd El-Ghani SF, Abdelfattah MY, Abou-Zeid AW, Ibrahim SH, Elshamaa MM (2023) Evaluation of the biocompatibility, antibacterial and anticancer effects of a novel nano-structured Fe–Mn-based biodegradable alloys in vitro study. Heliyon 9(11). https://doi.org/10.1016/j.heliyon.2023.e20932

Fântânariu M, Trincă LC, Solcan C et al (2015) A new Fe–Mn–Si alloplastic biomaterial as bone grafting material: In vivo study. Appl Surf Sci 352:129–139. https://doi.org/10.1016/J.APSUSC.2015.04.197

Feng Q, Zhang D, Xin C et al (2013) Characterization and in vivo evaluation of a bio-corrodible nitrided iron stent. J Mater Sci Mater Med 24:713–724. https://doi.org/10.1007/s10856-012-4823-z

Fiocchi J, Lemke JN, Zilio S, Biffi CA, Coda A, Tuissi A (2021) The effect of Si addition and thermomechanical processing in an Fe-Mn alloy for biodegradable implants: Mechanical performance and degradation behavior. Mater Today Commun 27:102447. https://doi.org/10.1016/j.mtcomm.2021.102447

Gao C, Peng S, Feng P, Shuai C (2017) Bone biomaterials and interactions with stem cells. Bone Res 5:1 5:1–33. https://doi.org/10.1038/boneres.2017.59

Gao C, Yao M, Shuai C, et al (2020) Advances in biocermets for bone implant applications. Bio-Design Manuf 3:4 3:307–330. https://doi.org/10.1007/S42242-020-00087-3

Geurtsen W (2002) Biocompatibility of dental casting alloys. Crit Rev Oral Biol Med 13:71–84. https://doi.org/10.1177/154411130201300108

Godec M, Kraner J, Skobir Balantič D, Paulin I, Drobne D, Kononenko V, Kocijan A, McGuiness P, Donik Č (2024) Bioresorbability dependence on microstructure of additively-manufactured and conventionally-produced Fe-Mn alloys. J Mater Res Technol 30:4881–4892. https://doi.org/10.1016/j.jmrt.2024.04.097

Gorejová R, Haverová L, Oriňaková R et al (2019) Recent advancements in Fe-based biodegradable materials for bone repair. J Mater Sci 54:1913–1947. https://doi.org/10.1007/s10853-018-3011-z

Hanas T, Sampath Kumar TS, Perumal G et al (2018) Electrospun PCL/HA coated friction stir processed AZ31/HA composites for degradable implant applications. J Mater Process Technol 252:398–406. https://doi.org/10.1016/J.JMATPROTEC.2017.10.009

Haverová L, Oriňaková R, Oriňak A et al (2018) An in vitro corrosion study of open cell Iron structures with PEG coating for bone replacement applications. Metals (Basel) 8:1–21. https://doi.org/10.3390/met8070499

Hermawan H, Alamdari H, Mantovani D, Dubé D (2008) Iron–manganese: new class of metallic degradable biomaterials prepared by powder metallurgy. Powder Metall 51:38–45. https://doi.org/10.1179/174329008X284868

Hermawan H, Dubé D, Mantovani D (2010a) Degradable metallic biomaterials for cardiovascular applications. In: Metals for biomedical devices. Elsevier Ltd, pp 379–404

Hermawan H, Dubé D, Mantovani D (2007) Development of degradable Fe-35Mn alloy for biomedical application. Adv Mat Res 15–17:107–112. https://doi.org/10.4028/www.scientific.net/AMR.15-17.107

Hermawan H, Purnama A, Dube D et al (2010b) Fe-Mn alloys for metallic biodegradable stents: degradation and cell viability studies. Acta Biomater 6:1852–1860. https://doi.org/10.1016/j.actbio.2009.11.025

Hočevar M, Donik Č, Paulin I, et al (2017) Corrosion on polished and laser-textured surfaces of An Fe–Mn biodegradable alloy. Materiali in Tehnologije 51:1037–1041. https://doi.org/10.17222/mit.2017.140

Hong D, Chou DT, Velikokhatnyi OI et al (2016) Binder-jetting 3D printing and alloy development of new biodegradable Fe-Mn-Ca/Mg alloys. Acta Biomater 45:375–386. https://doi.org/10.1016/j.actbio.2016.08.032

Hrubovčáková M, Kupková M, Džupon M, et al (2017) Biodegradable polylactic acid and polylactic acid/hydroxyapatite coated iron foams for bone replacement materials. Int J Electrochem Sci 12:11122–11136. https://doi.org/10.20964/2017.12.53

Huang S, Ulloa A, Nauman E, Stanciu L (2020) Collagen coating effects on Fe–Mn bioresorbable alloys. J Orthopaedic Res® 38:523–535. https://doi.org/10.1002/JOR.24492

Huang T, Cheng J, Bian D, Zheng Y (2016a) Fe–Au and Fe–Ag composites as candidates for biodegradable stent materials. J Biomed Mater Res B Appl Biomater 104:225–240. https://doi.org/10.1002/jbm.b.33389

Huang T, Cheng J, Zheng YF (2014) In vitro degradation and biocompatibility of Fe–Pd and Fe–Pt composites fabricated by spark plasma sintering. Mater Sci Eng C 35:43–53. https://doi.org/10.1016/j.msec.2013.10.023

Huang T, Cheng Y, Zheng Y (2016b) In vitro studies on silver implanted pure iron by metal vapor vacuum arc technique. Colloids Surf B Biointerfaces 142:20–29. https://doi.org/10.1016/j.colsurfb.2016.01.065

Huang T, Zheng Y (2016) Uniform and accelerated degradation of pure iron patterned by Pt disc arrays. Sci Rep 6:23627. https://doi.org/10.1038/srep23627

Huang T, Zheng Y, Han Y (2016c) Accelerating degradation rate of pure iron by zinc ion implantation. Regen Biomater 3:205–215. https://doi.org/10.1093/rb/rbw020

Hufenbach J, Wendrock H, Kochta F et al (2017) Novel biodegradable Fe–Mn-C-S alloy with superior mechanical and corrosion properties. Mater Lett 186:330–333. https://doi.org/10.1016/j.matlet.2016.10.037

Kraus T, Moszner F, Fischerauer S et al (2014) Biodegradable Fe-based alloys for use in osteosynthesis: outcome of an in vivo study after 52 weeks. Acta Biomater 10:3346–3353. https://doi.org/10.1016/j.actbio.2014.04.007

Lin WJ, Zhang DY, Zhang G et al (2016) Design and characterization of a novel biocorrodible iron-based drug-eluting coronary scaffold. Mater des 91:72–79. https://doi.org/10.1016/j.matdes.2015.11.045

Liu B, Zheng YF, Ruan L (2011) In vitro investigation of Fe30Mn6Si shape memory alloy as potential biodegradable metallic material. Mater Lett 65:540–543. https://doi.org/10.1016/j.matlet.2010.10.068

Mandal S, Ummadi R, Bose M et al (2019) Fe–Mn–Cu alloy as biodegradable material with enhanced antimicrobial properties. Mater Lett 237:323–327. https://doi.org/10.1016/j.matlet.2018.11.117

Montufar EB, Horynová M, Casas-Luna M et al (2016) Spark plasma sintering of load-bearing iron-carbon nanotube-tricalcium phosphate cermets for orthopaedic applications. JOM 68:1134–1142. https://doi.org/10.1007/S11837-015-1806-9/FIGURES/8

Nouri A, Wen C (2021) Noble metal alloys for load-bearing implant applications. Structural Biomaterials 127–156. https://doi.org/10.1016/B978-0-12-818831-6.00003-3

Oriňaková R, Gorejová R, Králová ZO, Oriňak A (2020) Surface modifications of biodegradable metallic foams for medical applications. Coatings 10. https://doi.org/10.3390/coatings10090819

Oriňaková R, Gorejová R, Macko J et al (2019) Evaluation of in vitro biocompatibility of open cell iron structures with PEG coating. Appl Surf Sci 475:515–518. https://doi.org/10.1016/j.apsusc.2019.01.010

Paul B, Kiel A, Otto M, Gemming T, Hoffmann V, Giebeler L, Kaltschmidt B, Hütten A, Gebert A, Kaltschmidt B, Kaltschmidt C (2024) Inherent antibacterial properties of biodegradable FeMnC (Cu) alloys for implant application. ACS Appl Bio Mater 7(2):839–852. https://doi.org/10.1021/acsabm.3c00835

Qi Y, Li X, He Y et al (2019) Mechanism of acceleration of iron corrosion by a polylactide coating. ACS Appl Mater Interfaces 11:202–218. https://doi.org/10.1021/acsami.8b17125

Rabeeh VPM, Hanas T (2022a) Enhancing biointerfacial properties of porous pure iron by gold sputtering for degradable implant applications. Mater Today Commun 31:103492. https://doi.org/10.1016/J.MTCOMM.2022.103492

Rabeeh VPM, Hanas T (2022) Progress in manufacturing and processing of degradable Fe-based implants: a review. Progress in Biomaterials 11:2 11:163–191. https://doi.org/10.1007/S40204-022-00189-4

Rabeeh VM, Rahim SA, Kinattingara Parambath S, Rajanikant GK, Hanas T (2023) Iron–gold composites for biodegradable implants: in vitro investigation on biodegradation and biomineralization. ACS Biomater Sci Eng 9:4255–4268. https://doi.org/10.1021/acsbiomaterials.3c00513

Rabeeh VPM, Surendramohan KS, Jyothis S et al (2024a) Fostering biomineralization and biodegradation: nano-hydroxyapatite reinforced iron composites for biodegradable implant application. Discov Mater 4:39. https://doi.org/10.1007/s43939-024-00113-6

Rabeeh VM, Surendramohan KS, Tharayil H (2024b) Bioactive Fe foam for degradable bone graft cages. Adv Eng Mater 26:2301416. https://doi.org/10.1002/adem.202301416

Rahim SA, Muhammad Rabeeh VP, Joseph MA, Hanas T (2021) Does acid pickling of Mg–Ca alloy enhance biomineralization? J Magn Alloys 9:1028–1038. https://doi.org/10.1016/J.JMA.2020.12.002

Reindl A, Borowsky R, Hein SB et al (2014) Degradation behavior of novel Fe/ß-TCP composites produced by powder injection molding for cortical bone replacement. J Mater Sci 49:8234–8243. https://doi.org/10.1007/s10853-014-8532-5

Sahu MR, Sampath Kumar TS, Chakkingal U, Dewangan VK, Doble M (2024) Enhancing the degradation rate and biomineralization nature of antiferromagnetic Fe-20Mn alloy by groove pressing. J Biomed Mater Res A. https://doi.org/10.1002/jbm.a.37711

Salama M, Vaz MF, Colaço R et al (2022) Biodegradable iron and porous iron: mechanical properties, degradation behaviour, manufacturing routes and biomedical applications. J Funct Biomater 13:72. https://doi.org/10.3390/jfb13020072

Schinhammer M, Gerber I, Hänzi AC, Uggowitzer PJ (2013a) On the cytocompatibility of biodegradable Fe-based alloys. Mater Sci Eng C 33:782–789. https://doi.org/10.1016/j.msec.2012.11.002

Schinhammer M, Hänzi AC, Löffler JF, Uggowitzer PJ (2010) Design strategy for biodegradable Fe-based alloys for medical applications. Acta Biomater 6:1705–1713. https://doi.org/10.1016/j.actbio.2009.07.039

Schinhammer M, Pecnik CM, Rechberger F et al (2012) Recrystallization behavior, microstructure evolution and mechanical properties of biodegradable Fe-Mn-C(-Pd) TWIP alloys. Acta Mater 60:2746–2756. https://doi.org/10.1016/j.actamat.2012.01.041

Schinhammer M, Steiger P, Moszner F et al (2013b) Degradation performance of biodegradable FeMnC(Pd) alloys. Mater Sci Eng C 33:1882–1893. https://doi.org/10.1016/j.msec.2012.10.013

Sharipova A, Gotman I, Psakhie SG, Gutmanas EY (2019) Biodegradable nanocomposite Fe–Ag load-bearing scaffolds for bone healing. J Mech Behav Biomed Mater 98:246–254. https://doi.org/10.1016/j.jmbbm.2019.06.033

Shuai C, Li Y, Yang Y et al (2016) Bioceramic enhances the degradation and bioactivity of iron bone implant. Mater Res Express 6:115401. https://doi.org/10.1088/2053-1591/ab45b9

Shuai C, Li Y, Yang Y et al (2019) Bioceramic enhances the degradation and bioactivity of iron bone implant. Mater Res Express 6:115401. https://doi.org/10.1088/2053-1591/ab45b9

Sikora-Jasinska M, Chevallier P, Turgeon S et al (2019) Understanding the effect of the reinforcement addition on corrosion behavior of Fe/Mg2Si composites for biodegradable implant applications. Mater Chem Phys 223:771–778. https://doi.org/10.1016/j.matchemphys.2018.11.068

Sun Y, Chen L, Liu N et al (2021) Laser-modified Fe–30Mn surfaces with promoted biodegradability and biocompatibility toward biological applications. J Mater Sci 56:13772–13784. https://doi.org/10.1007/S10853-021-06139-Y/FIGURES/9

Traverson M, Heiden M, Stanciu LA et al (2018) In vivo evaluation of biodegradability and biocompatibility of Fe30Mn alloy. Veterinary Comparative Orthopaedics and Traumatology 31:10–16. https://doi.org/10.3415/VCOT-17-06-0080

Trincă LC, Burtan L, Mareci D et al (2021) Evaluation of in vitro corrosion resistance and in vivo osseointegration properties of a FeMnSiCa alloy as potential degradable implant biomaterial. Mater Sci Eng C 118:111436. https://doi.org/10.1016/j.msec.2020.111436

Tripathi G, Pandey PM (2024) Study of compaction-free fabrication of topologically ordered functionally graded iron-hydroxyapatite-zinc biodegradable composite implants. J Mater Sci, 1–17.https://doi.org/10.1007/s10853-024-09786-z

Ulum MF, Arafat A, Noviana D et al (2014) In vitro and in vivo degradation evaluation of novel iron-bioceramic composites for bone implant applications. Mater Sci Eng C 36:336–344. https://doi.org/10.1016/j.msec.2013.12.022

Wang H, Zheng Y, Liu J et al (2017a) In vitro corrosion properties and cytocompatibility of Fe-Ga alloys as potential biodegradable metallic materials. Mater Sci Eng C 71:60–66. https://doi.org/10.1016/j.msec.2016.09.086

Wang S, Xu Y, Zhou J et al (2017b) In vitro degradation and surface bioactivity of iron-matrix composites containing silicate-based bioceramic. Bioact Mater 2:10–18. https://doi.org/10.1016/j.bioactmat.2016.12.001

Wegener B, Sievers B, Utzschneider S, et al (2011) Microstructure, cytotoxicity and corrosion of powder-metallurgical iron alloys for biodegradable bone replacement materials. In: Materials Science and Engineering B: Solid-State Materials for Advanced Technology. Elsevier B.V., pp 1789–1796

Wen Z, Zhang L, Chen C et al (2013) A construction of novel iron-foam-based calcium phosphate/chitosan coating biodegradable scaffold material. Mater Sci Eng C 33:1022–1031. https://doi.org/10.1016/j.msec.2012.10.009

Xu Z, Hodgson MA, Cao P (2015a) Microstructure and degradation behavior of forged Fe–Mn–Si alloys. Int J Mod Phys B 29. https://doi.org/10.1142/S0217979215400147

Xu Z, Hodgson MA, Cao P (2015b) A comparative study of powder metallurgical (PM) and wrought Fe–Mn–Si alloys. Mater Sci Eng A 630:116–124. https://doi.org/10.1016/j.msea.2015.02.021

Yusop AHM, Daud NM, Nur H et al (2015) Controlling the degradation kinetics of porous iron by poly(lactic-co-glycolic acid) infiltration for use as temporary medical implants. Sci Rep 5:11194. https://doi.org/10.1038/srep11194

Zhao YC, Tang Y, Zhao MC et al (2020) Study on Fe-xGO composites prepared by selective laser melting: microstructure, hardness, biodegradation and cytocompatibility. JOM 72:1163–1174. https://doi.org/10.1007/s11837-019-03814-z

Zheng YF, Gu XN, Witte F (2014) Biodegradable metals. Mater Sci Eng R Rep 77:1–34

Zhu S, Huang N, Shu H et al (2009) Corrosion resistance and blood compatibility of lanthanum ion implanted pure iron by MEVVA. Appl Surf Sci 256:99–104. https://doi.org/10.1016/j.apsusc.2009.07.082

Chapter 5
Biodegrdable Fe: Applications

5.1 Introduction

Biodegradable iron offers a compelling solution for various medical implant applications, primarily because of its favorable mechanical properties and biocompatibility. Biodegradable materials as a whole hold significant potential across a broad range of medical fields (Fig. 5.1). Based on current research, three primary areas stand out where clinical progress is particularly promising: bone implants, coronary stents, and tissue engineering scaffolds. While some biodegradable materials have already been integrated into medical practice, these technologies remain in their early stages of development. The degradable coronary stents and bone fixation devices have already been initially used in clinical treatments, demonstrating the practical benefits of this approach.

This chapter explores the various applications of biodegradable iron, with a focus on its use in cardiovascular, orthopedics and tissue engineering. This section will explore both in vivo and in vitro research, highlighting the positive aspects and challenges of using iron-based implants. These implants are engineered for sufficient structural support during tissue repair and gradually degrade and are absorbed by the body.

5.2 Cardiovascular Applications

Numerous cardiovascular applications predominantly emphasize the use of stents. Stenting, known clinically as percutaneous coronary intervention (PCI), has become a recognized technique for addressing obstructed coronary arteries (Garg and Serruys 2010). This treatment involves the delivery and placement of one or more stents within a constricted coronary artery via a catheter system. The catheter is introduced into the artery through a little incision, usually located in the arm or groin. Stents offer

© The Author(s), under exclusive license to Springer Nature Switzerland AG 2025   89
VP. Md. Rabeeh and T. Hanas, *Biodegradable Iron Implants: Development, Processing, and Applications*, SpringerBriefs in Materials,
https://doi.org/10.1007/978-3-031-82099-1_5

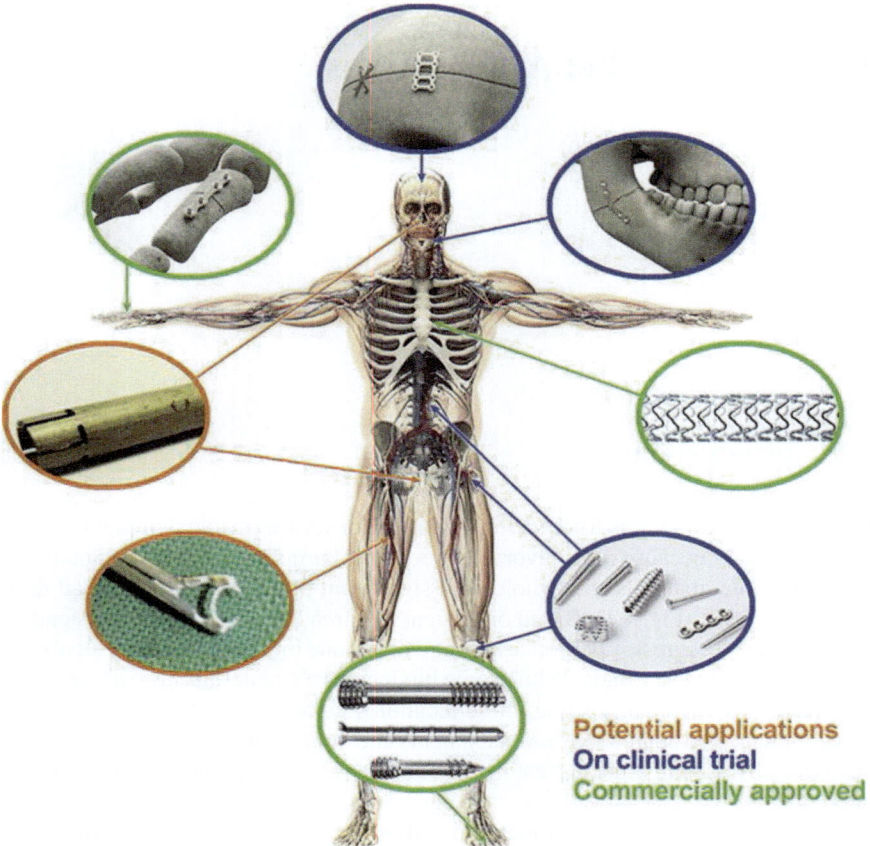

Fig. 5.1 Overview of various applications of biodegradble implants. Reprinted with permission of Elsevier from Han et al. (2019)

structural reinforcement by functioning as a mechanical scaffold, thereby mitigating early arterial recoil and late-stage vascular remodeling—two major limitations of conventional balloon angioplasty (Serruys et al. 1994; Fischman et al. 1994). PCI involves the disruption of arterial plaque and the dilation of the artery's diameter using high-pressure balloon inflation (Fig. 5.2). PCI possesses significant promise for enhancing patient outcomes and mitigating arterial thickening or hardening. This method is more easy and less invasive than coronary artery bypass graft surgery.

Stainless steel (SS) is commonly used for stents due to its favorable properties, but it has low radiopacity and is prone to pitting and crevice corrosion. Tantalum (Ta) provides excellent radiopacity and corrosion resistance, while Nitinol (a Ni–Ti alloy) features superelasticity and shape memory, though it can also suffer from corrosion issues (Korei et al. 2022). Co–Cr alloys offer high corrosion and wear resistance but have lower plasticity and workability than stainless steel. However, the use

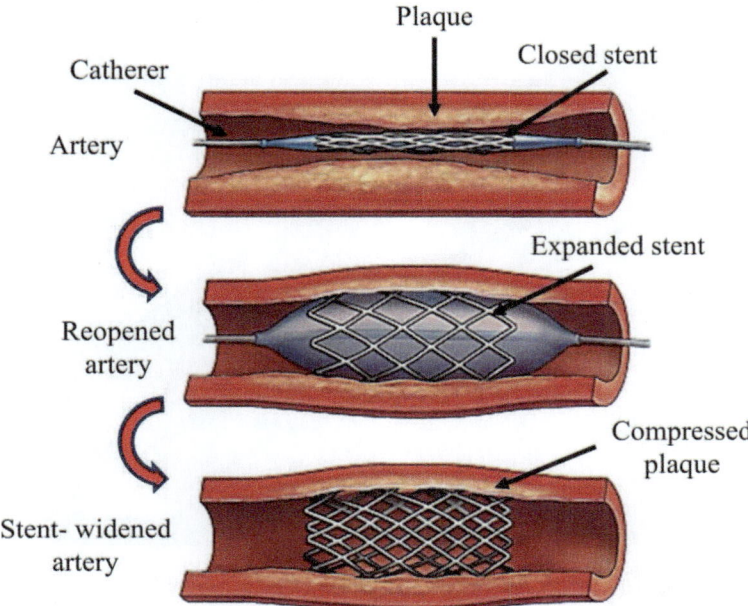

Fig. 5.2 Schematic illustration of percutaneous coronary intervention (PCI) or coronary angioplasty Reprinted with permission of Elsevier from Korei et al. (2022)

of permanent metallic stents has been linked to various challenges, such as persistent endothelial dysfunction, delayed re-endothelialization, increased risk of thrombosis, and prolonged local inflammation (Liu et al. 2023). In contrast, biodegradable vascular scaffolds represent a significant advancement in interventional cardiology, often referred to as the "fourth revolution" (Korei et al. 2022). These scaffolds offer numerous benefits, including their suitability for pediatric patients, eliminating the need for additional surgeries, reducing the risk of bleeding, and minimizing the chances of restenosis and late-stage thrombosis. Biodegradable metals are used in pure metals, alloys, and metal matrix composites for various cardio vascular application. The essential aspects in the design of BMs involve mechanical properties, including strength, hardness, elongation, and elastic modulus; chemical properties, such as biodegradability, ion release, absorbability, and pH behavior; physical properties like MRI compatibility, wettability, and radiopacity; and biological properties, which include biocompatibility, hemocompatibility, and osteoconductivity.

Among various BMs, Fe-based alloys have been widely studied and developed (Hermawan 2012, Peuster et al. 2006). Figure 5.3 shows the conventional stent made by SS and noval biodegradable Fe.

Nitrided Fe-based coronary scaffold developed by Lifetech Scientific features a sirolimus-eluting covering that accelerates corrosion rates via microenvironment acidification, resulting in complete absorption within 2–3 years (McLennan et al.

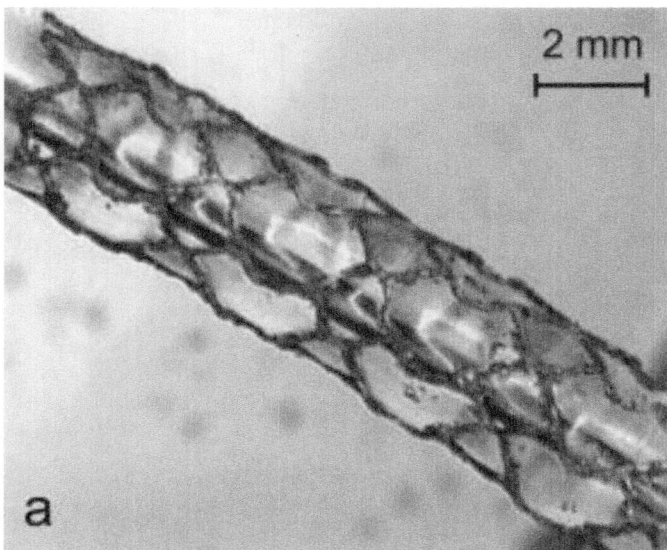

Fig. 5.3 Biodegradable stent made by Fe. Reprinted with permission of Elsevier from Hermawan (2010)

2024). Furthermore, studies indicate that iron stents demonstrate similar neointimal proliferation to conventional stainless steel stents, without inducing local toxicity or iron overload, hence affirming their appropriateness for therapeutic use (Zong et al. 2022). Additionally, innovative alloy compositions, such as Fe-10Mn-1Pd, have been examined to improve mechanical performance and degradation rates, illustrating the potential for customized designs that address particular clinical requirements (Kraus et al. 2014). These developments indicate a promising future for iron-based biodegradable stents in cardiovascular applications, with continued research aimed at enhancing their performance and clinical effectiveness.

5.2.1 Biosafety of Fe-Based Stents

The development of novel metallic resorbable stents demands a comprehensive evaluation of their biocompatibility throughout the degradation process. For clinical use, Fe-based stents must avoid releasing harmful degradation by-products, whether soluble or insoluble, and should not disrupt blood homeostasis or trigger prolonged inflammatory reactions. Considering that iron is inherently present in human tissues and blood (about 45–55 mg Fe/kg body weight), it has been proposed that the corrosion products of Fe-based stents will not induce systemic toxicity. Conversely, these by-products are anticipated to be metabolized and excreted through natural physiological mechanisms. Under aerobic conditions, iron experiences a redox transformation from Fe^{2+} to Fe^{3+}, characterized by a favorable redox potential of $+772$ mV. This oxidation reaction is pivotal in fundamental metabolic processes, rendering iron an indispensable metal for cellular activities.

The extracellular Fe^{3+}, due to its near insolubility, is complexed by particular iron-binding proteins such as transferrin (Tf), which aids in its transport to the cell membrane. The iron is transported into the endosomes by TfR1 receptor-mediated cellular absorption. Nonetheless, the plasma proteins in the body that sequester iron possess a finite capacity, and an accumulation of iron can be detrimental to cells and tissues. The deleterious effects of iron mostly stem from its capacity to stimulate free radical production. Moreover, the redox activity of iron can lead to the production of reactive oxygen species (ROS), which, at elevated concentrations, induce oxidative stress in cells. Consequently, it is essential to regulate the release of iron from degrading Fe-based stents to prevent excessive and rapid release, thereby avoiding toxicity and oxidative stress.

5.3 Orthopaedic Applications

The mechanical characteristics and biodegradability of Fe-based implants make them attractive options for orthopedic applications, especially bone tissue engineering. Iron (Fe) demonstrates superior strength and hardness, making it appropriate for load-bearing applications including screws, plates, and pins.

Despite its benefits, the slow degradation rate of Fe in physiological environments presents challenges for its use in bone healing. Research indicates that although Fe can offer sufficient mechanical support, its degradation must be precisely tuned to align with the pace of bone regeneration to guarantee that the implant does not exceed the duration of the healing process (Rabeeh and Hanas 2022). In vivo studies demonstrated that iron-based interference screws not only maintained high biomechanical performance but also enhanced bone volume and surface area in close proximity to the implant, indicating effective osteointegration (Tai et al. 2022).

Orthopedic screws are critical objects employed in orthopedic surgery to support and promote the healing of cracked or compromised bones. Their principal role is to consolidate bone fragments, reducing interstices and facilitating expedited healing. Engineered with precision these screws are generally fabricated from biocompatible materials like titanium or stainless steel, ensuring their compatibility with the body. There are several types of orthopedic screws, such as cortical screws for dense bone, cancellous screws for softer bone, and cannulated screws that enable accurate insertion over a guide wire. Different types of orthopedic screws currently in the markets are given Fig. 5.4. The selection of screw type is contingent upon the particular fracture features and the relevant anatomical place (Gefen 2002; Agarwal et al. 2022).

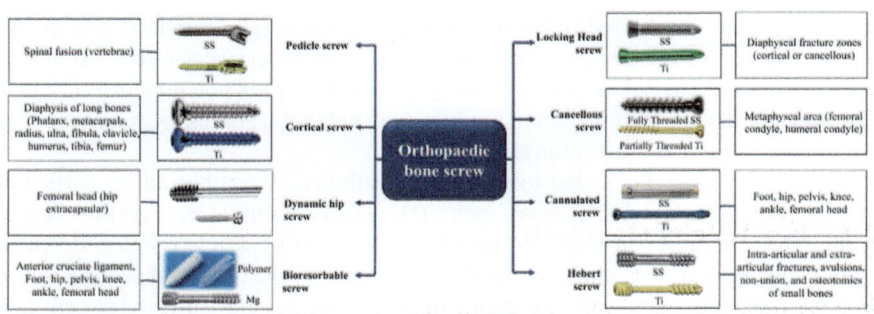

Fig. 5.4 Various types of bone screws used for different applications within the human body

Screw fixation is essential in orthopedic operations since it offers mechanical support to shattered bones. The design of orthopedic screws include self-tapping characteristics, enabling them to forge their own trajectory through the bone upon insertion, so minimizing surgical damage. Locking screws are significant because they create a fixed-angle construct when utilized with locking plates, hence improving stability in complicated fractures. The efficacy of screw fixation depends on parameters including thread design, length, and diameter, which must be meticulously chosen to provide good bone engagement and sufficient load distribution (Stahel et al. 2017).

Although conventional metal screws offer superior mechanical support, they often necessitate removal post-healing. This has prompted the investigation of biodegradable alternatives, such iron-based or polymeric screws, which can be assimilated by the body over time, so obviating the necessity for a secondary surgical procedure (Rabeeh and Hanas 2022).

5.4   Other Applications

5.4.1   Gastrointestinal Applications

In gastrointestinal (GI) treatments, Fe-based biodegradable implants are becoming a promising alternative to conventional approaches, providing significant advantages for both patients and physicians. Conventional staples and sutures employed in these operations frequently necessitate subsequent surgeries for removal, which can be invasive and elevate the chances of consequences, including infections, prolonged recovery periods, and increased medical costs. Iron-based biodegradable implants, such as staples, sutures, and clips, are engineered to offer essential mechanical support during tissue repair and then dissolve over time, thereby obviating the necessity for a secondary surgical intervention (Lu et al. 2024).

5.4.2 Urological Devices

The application of Fe-based biodegradable polymers in urology is highly promising. Urological implants, including stents utilized in the urinary system, typically necessitate removal upon the completion of their function, a procedure that can be both painful and costly. In contrast, Fe-based biodegradable stents offer crucial support for healing or fluid drainage and thereafter disintegrate naturally, obviating the necessity for a secondary removal surgery. Biodegradable urethral stents are one important application. These stents are frequently employed to address urethral blockages, which may occur due to scarring, trauma, or disorders such as benign prostatic hyperplasia (BPH). Conventional stents require removal when the obstruction is alleviated; however, biodegradable Fe-based stents provide a transient solution that dissolves post-healing (Ma et al. 2019). This method diminishes patient discomfort and mitigates the hazards linked to stent retrieval. Moreover, iron's corrosion characteristics in the urinary system—being less corrosive than in the gastrointestinal tract—render it an optimal candidate for these uses. The stent's progressive deterioration guarantees essential mechanical support for healing without necessitating additional surgical procedures (Waksman et al. 2008).

References

Agarwal R, Gupta V, Singh J (2022) Additive manufacturing-based design approaches and challenges for orthopaedic bone screws: a state-of-the-art review. J Braz Soc Mech Sci Eng 44:37. https://doi.org/10.1007/s40430-021-03331-8

Fischman DL, Leon MB, Baim DS et al (1994) A randomized comparison of coronary-stent placement and balloon angioplasty in the treatment of coronary artery disease. N Engl J Med 331(8):496–501

Garg S, Serruys PW (2010) Coronary stents: current status. J Am Coll Cardiol 56(10S):S42

Gefen A (2002) Optimizing the biomechanical compatibility of orthopedic screws for bone fracture fixation. Med Eng Phys 24(5):337–347. https://doi.org/10.1016/S1350-4533(02)00027-9

Han HS, Loffredo S, Jun I et al (2019) Current status and outlook on the clinical translation of biodegradable metals. Mater Today 23:57–71. https://doi.org/10.1016/j.mattod.2018.05.018

Hermawan H (2012) Biodegradable metals for cardiovascular applications. In: Biodegradable metals. SpringerBriefs in Materials. Springer, Berlin, Heidelberg. https://doi.org/10.1007/978-3-642-31170-3_3

Hermawan H, Dubé D, Mantovani D (2010) Developments in metallic biodegradable stents. Acta Biomater 6(5):1693–1697. https://doi.org/10.1016/j.actbio.2009.10.006

Korei N, Solouk A, Haghbin Nazarpak M, Nouri A (2022) A review on design characteristics and fabrication methods of metallic cardiovascular stents. Mater Today Commun 31:103467. https://doi.org/10.1016/j.mtcomm.2022.103467

Kraus T, Moszner F, Fischerauer S et al (2014) Biodegradable Fe-based alloys for use in osteosynthesis: Outcome of an in vivo study after 52 weeks. Acta Biomater 10(7):3346–3353. https://doi.org/10.1016/j.actbio.2014.04.007

Liu W, Wang X, Feng Y (2023) Restoring endothelial function: shedding light on cardiovascular stent development. Biomater Sci 11(12):4132–4150

Lu S, Wang P, Wang Q, Deng P, Yuan Y, Fu X, Yang Y, Tan L, Yang K, Qi X (2024) Biodegradable high-nitrogen iron alloy anastomotic staples: In vitro and in vivo studies. Bioact Mater 40:34–46. https://doi.org/10.1016/j.bioactmat.2024.06.005

Ma Z, Gao M, Na D, Li Y, Tan L, Yang K (2019) Study on a biodegradable antibacterial Fe–Mn–C–Cu alloy as urinary implant material. Mater Sci Eng C 103:109718. https://doi.org/10.1016/j.msec.2019.05.003

McLennan DI, Maldonado JR, Foerster SR et al (2024) Absorbable metal stents for vascular use in pediatric cardiology: progress and outlook. Front Cardiovasc Med 11:1410305. https://doi.org/10.3389/fcvm.2024.1410305

Peuster M, Beerbaum P, Bach FW, Hauser H (2006) Are resorbable implants about to become a reality? Cardiol Young 16(2):107–116. https://doi.org/10.1017/S1047951106000011

Rabeeh VPM, Hanas T (2022) Progress in manufacturing and processing of degradable Fe-based implants: a review. Progress Biomater 11:2 11:163–191. https://doi.org/10.1007/S40204-022-00189-4

Serruys PW, De Jaegere P, Kiemeneij F et al (1994) A comparison of balloon-expandable-stent implantation with balloon angioplasty in patients with coronary artery disease. N Engl J Med 331(8):489–495

Stahel PF, Alfonso NA, Henderson C et al (2017) Introducing the "Bone-Screw-Fastener" for improved screw fixation in orthopedic surgery: a revolutionary paradigm shift? Patient Saf Surg 11:6. https://doi.org/10.1186/s13037-017-0121-5

Tai CC, Huang YM, Liaw CK et al (2022) Biocompatibility and biological performance of additive-manufactured bioabsorbable iron-based porous interference screws in a rabbit model: a 1-year observational study. Int J Mol Sci 23(23):14626. https://doi.org/10.3390/ijms232314626

Waksman R, Pakala R, Baffour R et al (2008) Short-term effects of biocorrodible iron stents in porcine coronary arteries. J Interv Cardiol 21(1):15–20. https://doi.org/10.1111/j.1540-8183.2007.00319x

Zong J, He Q, Liu Y et al (2022) Advances in the development of biodegradable coronary stents: a translational perspective. Mater Today Bio 16:100368. https://doi.org/10.1016/j.mtbio.2022.100368

Chapter 6
Biodegrdable Fe: Summary & Future Prospective

6.1 Summary

The progress in tissue engineering necessitates that biomaterials display bio-functional properties. The future destiny for metallic implants is oriented towards the innovative application of biodegradable implants across multiple domains. The investigation of novel biodegradable metals is a fascinating area of research at forefront of biomaterials today. Biodegradable iron based implant, first introduced in 2001 with a stent prototype made from pure iron and tested on rabbits, have garnered the attention of biomaterial scientists. Several studies have been conducted leading up to the most major clinical investigation of absorbable magnesium stents and screws for cardiovascular and orthopedic applications. Nevertheless, a notable advancement has yet to be documented in iron-based implants. Despite almost two decades of development, a lack of comprehension continues to hinder the clinical use of this developing technology. To analyze and comprehend the relationship between the metal and its degradation product and the surrounding implantation site, as well as the in vivo degradation process and its kinetics, more in vitro and in vivo research is essential.

The reported studies suggest the potential of Fe-based technologies for biodegradable implants. However, no such product is introduced to the world market. The studies highlight that temporary implants must demonstrate a uniform degradation rate to prevent early failure. This largely relies on the degradation mechanism, which can be tailored by the altering de microstructure and composition. The research indicates that an appropriate combination of manufacturing methods and processing techniques, including alloying, microstructural modification, and surface modification, can facilitate the effective advancement of Fe-based biomedical materials.

Powder metallurgy (PM) and casting are the primary manufacturing techniques employed for developing Fe based biodegradable metals. The density and strength of the cast materials are higher than those of the powder metallurgically manufactured materials.

© The Author(s), under exclusive license to Springer Nature Switzerland AG 2025 97
VP. Md. Rabeeh and T. Hanas, *Biodegradable Iron Implants: Development, Processing, and Applications*, SpringerBriefs in Materials,
https://doi.org/10.1007/978-3-031-82099-1_6

A primary hurdle in the development of Fe-based implants is mitigating stress shielding, which arises when there is a substantial disparity between the elastic modulus of the implant and that of the adjacent bone. Iron-based materials generally exhibit a significantly greater elastic modulus than human bone, resulting in a disparity that can cause uneven load distribution. This discrepancy can impede natural bone regeneration and lead to bone resorption. Subsequent research should concentrate on optimizing the elastic characteristics of Fe-based materials to reduce stress shielding. Open-cell porous iron-based materials fabricated using powder metallurgy exhibit tailored degradation rate and mechanical properties comparable to those of human bone. Further research is required to refine pore morphology to closely resemble that of bone tissue, hence enhancing bioactivity and osseointegration. Methods like additive manufacturing (3D printing) and the integration of geometrically designed scaffolds also providing implants with mechanical properties more like to those of bone. 3D printing technology is a sophisticated and pioneering technique for creating precise, three-dimensional scaffolds and implants. Moreover, the 3D printing technique may be tailored to meet each patient's specific requirements, hence improving the effectiveness of the treatment procedure.

Moreover, controlling the rate of dissolution of Fe implants within the body is crucial to prevent fast degradation that might compromise implant integrity. A gradual, regulated degradation would guarantee the implant's functionality during the essential stages of tissue healing prior to its complete degradation, thereby avoiding damage to adjacent tissues.

Alloying significantly modified the microstructure and degradation characteristics of Fe-based materials among the processing procedures. Mn is the most commonly utilized alloying element in Fe for lowering its magnetic susceptibility. Non-traditional alloying elements such as Zn, Si, and Ag have also been used alongside Mn. The bulk of alloying elements expedited the deterioration rate during the in vitro degradation test. The use of noble elements including Cu, Pt, Pd, and Au has enhanced the rate of degeneration via galvanic coupling. The use of bioactive and biocompatible bioceramic phases enhanced osteointegration. However, more research is required to determine the toxicity of alloying elements in the physiological milieu as well as their methods of absorption and excretion. A comprehensive evaluation of the body's response to these novel implants merits investigation.

Multiple studies have concentrated on the surface modification of implant materials utilizing metallic, polymeric, and bioceramic substances. The use of polymeric and apatite coatings on porous Fe improved the biodegradation and biocompatibility of the materials. While the surface modifications resulted in considerable enhancement in bioactivity, its impact on mechanical properties requires further examination.

6.2 Future Prospective

To advance Fe-based biodegradable implants for clinical application, several critical research areas must be prioritized. Future research should concentrate on comprehending how alloying elements interact, as well as how their compositions and production procedures affect the rate of degradation and guarantee mechanical compatibility with bone tissue. To determine how these materials interact with biological systems over time, more in vitro and in vivo research are going to be necessary to examine the bio-interfacial characteristics. Furthermore, in order to accurately forecast long-term degradation behavior, it is imperative that shortcomings in present laboratory testing methodologies be addressed. Multidisciplinary research integrating materials science, bioengineering, and clinical studies is essential to expedite the transition of Fe-based biodegradable implants from the laboratory to clinical trials. In conclusion, although the advancement of Fe-based degradable implants is highly promising, it constitutes a long-term undertaking due to the intricate interactions with the physiological environment. However, Fe-based implants have the potential to soon become a dependable, minimally invasive option for temporary implant applications with further study into manufacturing technologies, materials processing, material compositions, and bioactivity.